· GROUP THERAPY IN TRANSACTIONAL ANALYSIS

Tangolo and Massi offer a complete manual for transactional analysis (TA)-based group therapy. *Group Therapy in Transactional Analysis* demonstrates the evolution of TA as a relational psychodynamic therapy rich in clinical experiences within both individual and group settings.

The authors outline how to select clients, which setting to provide, how to establish contracts, and which techniques to use during group sessions. The book includes a full assessment of research and theory, clearly demonstrating efficacy and taking into account neuroscientific studies on intersubjectivity and the social brain. This is combined with a practical approach which supports therapists from the very first steps to the analysis of more complex interpersonal dynamics and dream analysis in a group setting. Finally, future research directions are discussed, together with an overview of an experiment on online groups in the time of coronavirus.

This foundational text will be a key reference for therapists in training and professionals new to the principles of transactional analysis. It will also be of interest to students on psychotherapy training and clinical psychology courses.

Anna Emanuela Tangolo is Teaching and Supervising Transactional Analyst (psychotherapy), certified by the European Association for Transactional Analysis, and Director of the PerFormat Psychotherapy Specializing School in Pisa, Albenga, and Catania, Italy. She works as a psychotherapist in private practice with individuals, couples, and groups.

Anna Massi is Teaching and Supervising Transactional Analyst (psychotherapy) certified by the European Association for Transactional Analysis. She works in private practice with individuals, couples, and groups.

INNOVATIONS IN TRANSACTIONAL ANALYSIS: THEORY AND PRACTICE
Series Editor: William F. Cornell

This book series is founded on the principle of the importance of open discussion, debate, critique, experimentation, and the integration of other models in fostering innovation in all the arenas of transactional analytic theory and practice: psychotherapy, counseling, education, organizational development, health care, and coaching. It will be a home for the work of established authors and new voices.

TRANSACTIONAL ANALYSIS OF SCHIZOPHRENIA:
THE NAKED SELF
Zefiro Mellacqua

GROUPS IN TRANSACTIONAL ANALYSIS,
OBJECT RELATIONS, AND FAMILY SYSTEMS:
STUDYING OURSELVES IN COLLECTIVE LIFE
N. Michel Landaiche, III

CONTEXTUAL TRANSACTIONAL ANALYSIS:
THE INSEPARABILITY OF SELF AND WORLD
James M. Sedgwick

NEW THEORY AND PRACTICE OF TRANSACTIONAL
ANALYSIS IN ORGANIZATIONS: ON THE EDGE
S. J. van Poelje and Anne de Graaf

GROUP THERAPY IN TRANSACTIONAL ANALYSIS:
THEORY THROUGH PRACTICE
Anna Emanuela Tangolo and Anna Massi

www.routledge.com/Innovations-in-Transactional-Analysis-Theory-and-Practice/book-series/INNTA

GROUP THERAPY IN TRANSACTIONAL ANALYSIS

Theory through Practice

Anna Emanuela Tangolo and Anna Massi

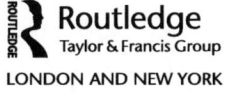

Routledge
Taylor & Francis Group

LONDON AND NEW YORK

First published 2022
by Routledge
4 Park Square, Milton Park, Abingdon, Oxon OX14 4RN

and by Routledge
605 Third Avenue, New York, NY 10158

Routledge is an imprint of the Taylor & Francis Group, an informa business

British Library Cataloguing-in-Publication Data
A catalogue record for this book is available from the British Library

Library of Congress Cataloging-in-Publication Data
Names: Tangolo, Anna Emanuela, author. | Massi, Anna, author.
Title: Group therapy in transactional analysis : theory through practice / Anna Emanuela Tangolo and Anna Massi.
Description: Milton Park, Abingdon, Oxon ; New York, NY : Routledge, 2022. | Series: Innovations in transactional analysis | Includes bibliographical references and index.
Identifiers: LCCN 2021048567 | ISBN 9781032104836 (hardback) | ISBN 9781032104812 (paperback) | ISBN 9781003215547 (ebook)
Subjects: LCSH: Group psychotherapy. | Transactional analysis.
Classification: LCC RC488 .T36 2022 | DDC 616.89/152—dc23/eng/20211117
LC record available at https://lccn.loc.gov/2021048567

ISBN: 978-1-032-10483-6 (hbk)
ISBN: 978-1-032-10481-2 (pbk)
ISBN: 978-1-003-21554-7 (ebk)

DOI: 10.4324/9781003215547

Typeset in Times New Roman
by Apex CoVantage, LLC

CONTENTS

CONTENTS

FOREWORD

William F. Cornell

With the publication of *Group Therapy in Transactional Analysis*, Anna Emanuela Tangolo and Anna Massi draw upon their decades of experience working together in therapy, supervision, and training groups to present a compelling and comprehensive accounting of contemporary TA group therapy.

This book comes 70 years after Eric Berne's publication of *Transactional Analysis in Psychotherapy* in which he grounded his theory and methods within the context of group therapy. This represented a radical break in his psychoanalytic training which had valorized the analytic dyad and the unconscious dynamics of intrapsychic conflict. His innovative emphasis on groups resulted in rejection by the psychoanalytic societies of the time. However, Berne sustained his interest in group life, referring to transactional analysis as a "social psychiatry" that constituted the study of people in their relations to one another and the wider social world. Each of first three books (1961, 1963, and 1966) was focused on groups and life within groups. With his characteristic humor, Berne suggested that the validation of therapeutic change was not so much in the eyes and satisfactions of the therapist but "in the resultant, independently observed changes in the behavior with intimates who have not been exposed to psychotherapy" (1961, p. 165), that is, in the real and ordinary world of the patients.

For Berne, the objective of group treatment was to carry the patients through the analysis of ego state functioning, transactions, games, and scripts so as to attain "social control," Berne's term for the capacity to use one's Adult ego state for self-awareness and conscious choice. Berne's premise – one shared by Tangolo and Massi – was that the diversity and dynamics of group membership mirrored the demands and unpredictability of life among others and, therefore, evoked patterns of defense (games and scripts) more rapidly than in individual psychotherapy. His goals were, in a sense rather modest, in fostering "improved social experiences [that] will lead to a diminution of archaic distortions and anxieties, with some relief of symptoms which is predictable, controllable, and intelligible to the patient as well as the therapist" (1961, p. 165). He saw group treatment as sometimes setting the ground for more intensive, psychoanalytic treatment. Berne himself often worked with patients in groups and then in individual psychoanalysis on the couch. As is evidenced in the pages of this book, transactional analytic group treatment has now evolved to the point that a move to the analytic couch is no longer seen as necessary to address the more entrenched and vulnerable patterns of needs and defenses.

In this volume, Tangolo and Massi ground their approach to group therapy in Berne's theories and methods but extend the depth and breadth of group treatment far beyond the reach described in Berne's own approach. While Berne's emphasis was on the cathexis of the Adult ego state and fostering of cognitive awareness, Tangolo and Massi see the group as a context and container within which regression, sometimes quite severe, can be welcomed, received, and transformed through intensity of here-and-now experiences within the group matrix. The group, in their eyes, has the essential functions to unsettle, evoke, contain, and reflect upon intense (and often unexpected) states of projection and disturbance, central to the resolution of persistent, unconscious troubled states of being within the Child ego state.

In Chapter 1, Tangolo and Massi ask, "Why the group?" – a question that they answer and illustrate in a multitude of ways throughout the pages of this book. In this chapter, they frame the group as a context within which patients (and therapists) situate themselves within a process of building a "social brain," such that

> the group setting and the cognitive nature of therapeutic operations together with the regressive and oneiric atmosphere – the latter of which facilitates the expression of transference processes and a deep reorganization of the self – constitute a truly rich wealth of experiences for a relevant psychodynamic psychotherapy, one that nurtures intersubjectivity and the We.

Throughout this book, the authors offer vivid examples of the impact and therapeutic opportunities afforded through the immediacy of emotional encounters within the group in the here-and-now. They argue, "In group, emotions are not recounted [after the fact] as in individual therapy, but they are directly experienced in the here-and-now because the presence of other members is a threat in and of itself."

Following Berne's sudden death in 1970 at 60 years of age, groups remained a central mode of treatment through the 1970s, although gradually losing emphasis among many of the following generations of TA psychotherapists. Attention became increasingly focused on individual psychotherapy, especially with the onset of relational models which have tended to focus on the dyad, grounded in the mother/infant dyad, and working through the transference/countertransference dynamics. Groups have, nonetheless, continued to be central in transactional analysis counseling, education, and organizational consultation, as well as in psychotherapy training and supervision. In the decades since Berne's death, changes and challenges to TA group models have been given voice in the *Transactional Analysis Journal*. *Group Therapy in Transactional Analysis* brings together these diverse voices from the *TAJ* into a comprehensive and integrative whole.

Tangolo and Massi re-situate group psychotherapy back at the heart of transactional analysis. This book is not only an elucidation of contemporary TA but also a rich and stimulating integration of TA with neurobiological and psychoanalytic perspectives.

The personal introductions and opening chapters of this book set group life and group treatment in a deeply human, humane, and historical frame. The midsection of the book then approaches the practicalities of forming and running groups, delineating such procedures as the selection of members, the contractual agreements, the physical settings, and termination, all of which are illustrated with case examples. The authors then undertake a re-examination of Berne's work and extend TA group psychotherapy into such areas as working with dreams, personality disorders, and depressive and bipolar states – territories that were not addressed by Berne.

In my own writing, I have returned again and again to a re-examination of Berne's writings. As is so often the case with the iconoclastic and disquieting innovators of new systems, their work often gets systematized and homogenized such that the original depth of thought and creative passions are lost. I have often sought to revive and re-present the depth and conflicted creativity of Berne's writings. In a similar spirit and fashion, Tangolo and Massi return to central concepts of Berne's group theories – deconfusion, therapeutic operations, and the group imago – re-presenting and revitalizing these fundamental concepts and procedures. While I found that this book is fascinating from beginning to end, these were the chapters that excited me the most. They take up Berne's concepts, bring new life and depth to them, and make them alive on the page through clinical examples. Throughout the book, their extensive use of case examples brings theory and practice alive for the reader.

As the book draws to a close, Tangolo and Massi offer an extended glimpse into a typical group. To say an "extended glimpse" may seem quite contradictory – how can a "glimpse" be "extended"? They bring to life 15 minutes of a group session, demonstrating how 15 minutes of real time in a group "extends" into the past and toward the future, capturing many hours of psychic time.

Rather paradoxically, much of this book was being crafted during the period of time when both time and place seemed to become frozen in place – the Covid-19 pandemic. Suddenly, like all of us, it was no longer possible to meet in person. Although our social, family, and group lives could not stop, they were suddenly, dramatically altered, as, in their words, "the pandemic has plunged us: collective fears, generalized anxiety, diffidence and need to trust, connect and belong." Tangolo and Massi offer a rich and optimistic reflection on the possibilities and limitations of groups working via screens.

As a therapist, supervisor, and trainer, *Group Therapy in Transactional Analysis* will not be sitting idly on my book shelves. It will become a well-worn favorite resource for my own work.

PREFACE

Personal evocations: How two group therapists are born

When we started writing this book, we already had many common experiences of clinical activity and training for psychotherapists in transactional analysis. Our work was always a collaboration and open exchange, and when we thought about writing a handbook on group therapy, we imagined it to be like the adventure and the journey of "two 70s girls" who, in the process of becoming adults, have accompanied many people in their growth.

In this preface, we would like to tell you something very intimate and personal, the same things we talked about when we told each other the reasons why we fell in love with group work. Please accept our offering as a sign of trust, for from this exchange is born the most personal and emotional part of our work.

Anna Emanuela

I am coming from the outside, where it is cold and rainy. I know the room will be warm and I will be able to dry myself off. I need warmth and to feel understood, to be surrounded by people lending me strength and comfort. What I am feeling right now is associated with far-away memories, the family kitchen on a winter's night, with wood burning in the stove, a pot on the fire and everyone there, mum helping us with our homework, and dad cleaning the mushrooms gathered in the forest. The cat sleeps on a chair, there is warmth, safety, and us children are drawing in our notebooks with the colors of the much-awaited spring.

Another group scene is in our farm at Cepponero, my grandparents' house. Another fire burns, lighting up the room, my aunt reading fairy tales to us girls and everyone else running around us doing things.

The summer scenario of the group is in the garden, under the stars, among the chirping of the crickets and a darkness that is reassuring because animated by laughter and benevolent presences.

Once more, the group is the reunion of all my cousins in Lecce for Christmas or Ferragosto, the games with my friends in the attic and in the woods.

For me, groups are always associated with pictures of warmth, affection, nourishment, pleasure, and fun. It may be for this reason that I am mostly a group therapist and love working in group even with my colleagues. These first images

xiv

have represented a guide which led me to turn toward ever more complex groups, such as those in school, politics, associated work, the scientific community, and conventions.

The more the world of groups became complex in my life, the more I needed to also detach myself, walk my own path, alone. However, as my parents always say, I have always done that. In my family, I was famous for my ability as a little girl to lose myself in a book even when I was in the same room with the others, and as a teenager to disappear in the woods for an entire day.

For me, the secret of life is knowing how to appropriately mix the times and spaces of solitude with the times and spaces of intimacy and crowdedness. Even now, at almost 60 years old, I look for days of silence and disconnection from everyone as precious moments of regeneration. The very time of sleep is a regenerating withdrawal, even if, at times, I find waiting for me in my dreams the same crowd I leave behind during the day and the same feelings of concern I try to shake off during the night's rest.

In therapy groups, I often see these two needs: the coming together for warmth and the need to detach myself and go my own way. The temporal rhythm of the periodical meeting pushes toward this exercise: first I get closer, getting in touch with people through transactional exchanges, seeking intimacy, then I differentiate myself from others' thoughts and emotions and put some distance, I define myself in difference with them, and I leave to find me alone with myself.

This exercise is very good for us because it makes us flexible, capable of getting closer and away, of feeling the bond in absence as well as the difference in presence. It is an exercise that should allow us to become more defined as individuals, more intimate with others, and more intersubjective in our reasoning: meaning, in the end, more profoundly human and mature.

The danger of an excess of proximity lies in group conformism, in the symbiotic relationships which lead us to regress to the pack or dependent sect mentality.

The danger of an excess of individualism pushes us toward a pathological narcissism and egotism which lead us to see others as objects to dominate, to use at our leisure, and to our ends.

Finding a healthy balance of interdependence is the result of a long journey of growth and maturation in a society as complex as ours, in which everyone should keep working on their personal growth for the entirety of their lives.

Anna Massi

I have always loved traveling. When I was a kid, I used to look forward to the summer holidays in my mum's parents' house, in the green of the Marchigian hills. From their house of stone, I could admire the vast golden fields of wheat, and far way I could catch a glimpse of the many shades of blue of the sea.

Then, when I was a teenager, I started to go on trips with my friends. We would often travel by train or hitchhike, in part to save money, in part because risk and adventure excited us. With a very low budget, we visited many places in Italy and

Europe, we managed to speak in languages we did not know very well, helped by intonation, looks, and gestures. We were fueled by an indefinite curiosity and we travelled along itineraries unknown to mass tourism. I have indelible memories of these trips and the encounters that took place during that time, with boys and girls from other countries and cultures: memories of windows of freedom.

During my university years, I started a different kind of journey, that of analysis, a journey which would go on for the rest of my life, interspersed with interruptions and reprisals, and accompanied by training in different schools of psychotherapy: first the psychoanalytical approach, then psychosynthesis, and finally transactional analysis.

I could compare this new journey to the path of the wanderer. When you walk on foot, you are not attached to a chair, lost in the frenzy of work, but you become master of a time that stretches on. The eyes of the wanderer travel through boundless spaces, rest on details, and spur emotions, thoughts, and bodily sensations. The body participates in the events of the journey, perceives the uneven ground and the blocked roads, and meets the grassy fields of childhood, while its feet decide the pace and trace the path.

"Wanderer, there is no road, the road is made by walking" recite the words of the beautiful poem by Antonio Machado titled "Wanderer." And this road I keep building together with my fellow travelers: friends, colleagues, therapists, supervisors, clients, and students. It is a road we "make" by walking together, our steps walking the line of our past, present, and future: the events of the past emerge in our memory to find a place and dignity in the present, as well as to offer an impulse of change to the future. It is not the emergence of past memories that fosters transformation, but the act of sharing these memories with others, since this act of sharing becomes collective memory.

I like to think of the group, whatever its form, as a band of wanderers of the mind, minds in motion, always changing perspectives thanks to the different points of view they acquire from others. Thoughts in motion, in evolution, which at times convey emotional sparks, expressing vague ideas and sensations, and other times become more solid and assume more definite shapes, but always seek new maps and new territories to explore.

And the journey goes on.

ACKNOWLEDGMENTS

This book has a long history and involves many people to whom we would like to express our gratitude. A book on groups is born out of many group exchanges, especially at PerFormat, the training school we founded and to which we are associated.

Thus, there are many associates, colleagues, and work groups that inspired us and that we want to thank. Our first debt of gratitude goes to the group atmosphere at PerFormat, in which we are always pursuing an "ecology of social relationships" – in the words of our associate Franco Bertozzi. To him, we are also extremely grateful for the support, encouragement, and the photography he graciously donated for our cover.

Thanks to Marina Zazo and Francesca Vignozzi, vivid and open minds, with whom we constantly share the passion for education and the exchanges of thoughts; together with them, Andrea Guerri, Patrizia Vinella, Pinuccia Casalegno, Graziella Cavanna, and Loredana Paradiso have an important role in fostering the scientific preparation of our students and discussing with us the themes we have treated in the book.

Our thoughts also go to Michele Novellino, one of our teachers and supervisors, who made us meet: it is in his training group that our passion for groups was born.

Our gratitude is particularly heartfelt for William Cornell, who was instrumental in guiding our work in research and innovation.

An enormous thank also goes to Paolo Migone, always generous and ready to offer us his invaluable support during conventions and clinical supervisions.

A particular thank to the colleagues of the research group, who are always committed to create a bridge between research, clinical practice, and training.

We are deeply grateful to Silvia Rosa, who went through every single page of this book with her keen eye, in an effort to make our ideas as coherent and easy to understand as possible.

Special thanks to Martina Del Romano for the English translation of the book, which took place at the same time as the writing of the Italian manuscript, and which made us think in a more open and global way, imagining readers from different countries and cultures. A big thanks also goes to Katie Randall,

ACKNOWLEDGMENTS

Editorial Assistant, and Alexis O'Brien, Editor of the English translation for Routledge and Rajalakshmi Ramesh for project managing the title.

To our students of the training school goes our utmost gratitude for the motivation to write and publish, fueled by our desire to be of help to their journey.

Finally, to our clients, thanks for teaching us every day how to be therapists.

And, looking back deeply into our past, a very special acknowledgment to our families, who taught us how to be in group, and to our sisters, Elena and Claudia, the first people with whom we shared time, love, and the world.

Anna Emanuela Tangoloe Anna Massi
Pisa, 2021

INTRODUCTION

The idea for this book was born several years ago, when we started sharing the reasons behind the efficacy of group therapy also with regard to the most severe of pathologies and talking about the influence of interpersonal neurobiology studies on emotional regulation in therapy groups.

Nowadays, much has changed since Berne wrote *Principles of Group Treatment*. Pathologies are not the same as back then, and conditions such as the narcissist or borderline personality disorders, which allow for a limited capacity of authentic involvement in social relationships, need spaces of healing that are oriented toward not only a reduction of the symptoms but also an improvement of these people's abilities to commit to healthier and more gratifying relationships.

Our book aims to describe these changes and present the techniques acquired in our work with transactional analysis psychodynamic groups, through a continuous dialectic process between theory and clinical practice.

What follows is an overview of the book's structure and contents.

Chapter 1 centers on interpersonal neurobiology, explaining how our brain molds itself in a relational context and how neuroplasticity intensifies within environments that provide syntonized interpersonal relationships. It is through stimulation from the child's caregivers that the brain becomes mind, meaning that it acquires the ability to read and interpret others' mental states as well as their own, a skill that Fonagy and colleagues call *mentalization*. The brain is a social organ developing and ripening thanks to our relationships with others and this chapter describes all the ways in which group therapy offers a reparative experience, promoting interpersonal learning and change, especially in people who experienced situations of isolation, emotional negligence, stress, and trauma in their childhood. Having a clear vision of the mind and understanding how to alter its functioning represent essential steps to be taken in order to lead our clients on a path to improved well-being.

Chapter 2 proposes a historical-developmental analysis of group theory starting from authors such as LeBon and Freud until the most recent developments related to the interpersonal approach, which shares many elements with transactional analysis, since it mainly takes into consideration interpersonal relationships and transactions within the group setting. The authors covered in this chapter are

1   DOI: 10.4324/9781003215547-1

connected with the field of psychoanalysis and many of their names can be found in Berne's *Principles of Group Treatment*.

The basic approaches we can identify in the historical development are three:

> The group is used as setting for individual therapy, where the therapist works one at a time with each client, denying any psychological specificity to the group as a whole.
>
> The group as a whole is the object of treatment and the therapist interacts with it as if it were a single individual.
>
> The interpersonal approach, the most widespread and the one we will find more often in the next chapters, allows clients to develop a better awareness of their maladaptive personal interactions and create new ways to understand and participate in the relational exchanges with fellow group members.

Chapter 3 further explores the interpersonal approach by taking an in-depth look at the factors that play a role within a well-functioning group, considering in particular the therapeutic factors described by Yalom. How does group psychotherapy help clients? This is the question this chapter seeks to give an answer to, in order to provide a regulating principle that therapists might use in the application of strategies and tactics that are most likely to implement efficacy in group therapy. Each therapeutic factor, from altruism to group cohesion, is connected to the main characteristics of the transactional analysis therapy group, especially to script decisions and beliefs about oneself and others. Factors tied to interpersonal learning and cohesion will be explored in depth in subsequent chapters of the book. These are complex and wide factors which are based on distorted images originating from relationships with past significant others, and the therapeutic alliance, both closely tied with positive outcomes to the treatment.

If Chapter 3 poses the question *How does group psychotherapy help clients?*, Chapter 4 asks: *How does the brain change through group therapy?* The clients' parts that are tied to trauma are activated by the stimuli of life in a therapy group and are often guided by implicit responses of a traumatic nature; clients might feel threatened and react with responses which correspond to the basic assumptions described in Chapter 2 in accordance with Bion's thought: fight-flight, dependency, and pairing. Understanding the neuroscientific principles, the way in which interpersonal relationships mold the brain might help group therapists to lower the chance of such maladaptive responses in clients and improve their emotional regulation. In this chapter, we identify those methods of group interactions which facilitate neuroplasticity, sustain neural integration, and lead to the development of more fulfilling relationships and improved group cohesion. When the implicit neural networks are activated in group, the latter, supported by the therapist, is able to amplify the syntonic feelings and, consequently, strengthen any possible reparations.

In order for the group to work as a safe space, it is necessary to proceed toward an accurate client selection and a good group composition. This is the main topic of Chapter 5, which presents the most recent studies regarding participation in therapy groups, as well as criteria of exclusion and inclusion. Exclusion criteria are related to the diagnosis and to some particular situations which characterize certain people's lives; as for inclusion criteria, group therapy has proven especially effective for those pathologies in which clients have troubles establishing intimate and gratifying relationships. The chapter also tackles the client's preparation to group therapy. Such preparation will have to take place during individual therapy with the group's conductor, who will provide the client with guidelines in order for them to make the most of their therapeutic experience. With respect to group composition, we compare the therapy group to a social microcosm, thus the more the group's structure is heterogeneous – in regard to both the different diagnostic classifications and the categories of age, gender, profession, and education – the more the chances its members will have to develop new learning opportunities.

Chapter 6 is dedicated to the setting, the rules, and the ethical principles regulating the relationship between members. Rules are not fixed but based on the European Association for Transactional Analysis (EATA) ethical code, which is inspired by the principles expressed in the *Universal Declaration of Human Rights*: respect, empowerment, protection, responsibility, and effort in the relationship. The therapist's duty is not exclusively tied to the non-violation of ethical norms, but on proactive actions aimed at facilitating the creation of a space of reflection where to foster a respect of opinions, beliefs, and value systems held by other members. The chapter also tackles the matter of combining group therapy with individual sessions every other week, or adding a weekly group therapy session after a period of individual therapy. Other themes are: relationships between members outside the group session, absences, lateness, payment, and the structuring of time.

Chapter 7 takes an in-depth look at the therapeutic alliance and the ways in which it may become a therapeutic influence on members. Group cohesion, one of the therapeutic factors discussed in Chapter 3, coincides with the relationship in individual therapy, but, unlike the latter, here it emerges as a wider and more complex concept. The therapeutic contract, which we have deemed contractual alliance, is the first step toward the activation of group cohesion. In this stage, treatment expectations are analyzed and a concrete structure for the setting is established. The contract involves the responsibility each member takes on to act sincerely and spontaneously, in order to develop a sense of belonging and take full advantage of the attraction the group exerts on its members. Alliances are often unstable in time and suffer incessant ruptures and resolutions, so we provide some guidelines on how to deal with such ruptures and further improve cohesion within the group.

Chapter 8 grapples with decontamination, meaning all type of interventions shedding light on the clients' cognitive structure. These interventions facilitate the emergence of problems and changes that need to be faced in order to reach the goals established in the contractual alliance. It is a stage that precedes deconfusion and clears up the pathological interactions between Parent, Adult, and Child.

The aim is to obtain an integrated Adult, free of the influence of unprocessed past experiences that remained fixed in both Child and Parent. We describe the qualms to group participation in terms of contaminations expressed through beliefs such as: *groups are dangerous, others will deem me inadequate*, or *I will be ignored and ridiculed because my problems are worthless to others*. When clients express their doubts aloud to the group, they receive meaningful feedback by fellow members and therapist, which helps them operate a distinction between their own pathogenic beliefs and the need for authentic relationships, thus decontaminating the Adult. Chapters 10 and 11 will delve into a description of the therapist's preferred methods of intervention in transforming of these beliefs.

Chapter 9 centers around deconfusion and introduces new material reflecting the progress made by transactional analysis in resolving the impasse that paralyzes clients' intrapsychic and relational lives. The chapter starts with a clarification of the concepts of script, confusion, and deconfusion, and later delves into the question of the transformation of the group's archaic decision in building a new narrative of self free from the shackles of script beliefs: A shared and collective narrative which allows the client to reconfigure their own position in the world through a new process of mirroring in the therapist and fellow members. Deconfusion work in group favors transference analysis thanks to the spontaneous contact with the most primitive aspects of each member's mind as well as the group mind. The individual and collective nature intersect through the creation of a network of interactions that support members' inner emotions.

Chapter 10 discusses the basic techniques suggested by Berne in *Principles of Group Treatment* in relation to therapeutic operations. These are specific transactional stimuli that the therapist offers the client in order to work on decontamination and deconfusion. The first six operations (interrogation, specification, confrontation, explanation, illustration, and confirmation) refer to decontamination, while the last two (interpretation and crystallization) to deconfusion. All interventions are aimed at producing change during group sessions and must be employed along with the therapist's empathic and careful listening skills. Their goal is to improve clients' awareness and create a space of reflection in which the past becomes recognizable and, as such, creates deep bonds between members, who become able to spontaneously open up to future perspectives. The chapter ends with the description of interventions at the hands of the therapist's Parent (support, reassurance, persuasion, and exhortation), operating on the Child ego state, and the bull's eye transaction which hits all three of the client's ego states.

Chapter 11 continues in the exploration of techniques, in this case the more advanced ones. When we talk about group therapy, we are facing extremely complex processes involving our being with ourselves in the world and our being with the other, that which is different from us, the stranger, the unknowable, but also that who is similar to us, with whom we share familiar aspects. For this reason, group processes require a specific set of techniques and skills. We start from the analysis of time structuring within a therapy group and then move on to the directing style to adopt in order to manage the thick and intricate network of relationships: When is it appropriate to let things happen and when instead is it necessary to take action so as to let the exchanges between members come to the surface? There is no perfect recipe to answer these questions, and it is mostly the psychotherapist's capacity to tolerate uncertainty that influences the therapeutic process, offering the possibility to accompany clients through their hardships on equal footing, abandoning all pretense of fixed certainties and illusions of life coaching.

Chapter 12 deals with the *group imago* and the processes of change that are involved in the different stages of its development. The group imago is a concept described by Berne as a mental image that group members and therapist have of the group experience in time, from the moment it starts until the very end. It is important to lead each member to the evolution of their personal imago to more advanced stages of development. The *provisional imago* corresponds to the individual image that is formed before joining the group. This imago changes into a second phase of development, the *provisional imago*, when the first contacts between members are established. When the interactions between members increase through the emergence of conflicts and games, the provisional imago transforms in *operative imago*. In the fourth phase, the group is more coherent and the deepest themes tied to the script start to surface: this phase is the *secondarily adjusted imago*. The fifth stage, the *clarified group imago*, corresponds to the end of therapy and the elaboration of detachment.

In Chapter 13, we analyze the parallelism between games and enactments according to transactional analysis, as well as the processes of transference and countertransference. Games theory saw many changes from Berne until today, and new in-depth studies push toward a redefinition of the nature of the therapeutic relationship even in group therapy. The therapist becomes an active observer and influences what they see, so their countertransference is crucial for the understanding of group dynamics, since they are situated within the transference–countertransference matrix. Enactments and games between clients and therapist reactivate the original traumas and lead to a power struggle between members to overcome others. Processing enactments allows clients to integrate the dissociated elements in order to build an integrated and differentiated identity while developing group cohesion and intimacy. At the end of the chapter, we take a brief look at the therapist's countertransference responses and members' lateral transferences with respect to specific personality disorders.

Chapter 14 examines dreamwork, through different cultural frameworks, in the developmental stages of the group process. Dream narration is analyzed in relation to the development of group imago. The mode of analysis is explorative and requires the creation of a space ready to contain and embrace all meaning produced by group members through the expression of free associations. In particular, we describe some of the dreams narrated and analyzed in group settings, linking them to imago analysis and to the way any alterations to this image emerge through the processes of decontamination and deconfusion. Communicating and sharing dreams lead to the exploration of new territories in which it is possible for clients to free themselves from old prejudices and enrich their inner and interpersonal world. All group members, even the quietest ones, participate in developing a new narration of the dream and it feels like everyone is contributing to the common good.

Chapter 15, on personality disorders, describes the most apt modes of intervention with clients suffering from such disorders, especially when it comes to the narcissistic and borderline structure of personality. Studies on long-term psychodynamic group psychotherapy proved that therapeutic groups offer many opportunities to clients with personality disorders. These clients are characterized by dysfunctional and pervasive traits involving different areas of the affective, cognitive, behavioral, and interpersonal functioning, such that compromise all of their relationships. In group, such clients tend to activate dramatic relational patterns which cast the therapist and fellow members in the role of Rescuer/Persecutor and themselves in the role of Victim/Persecutor. To them, being part of a therapy group means belonging to the interpersonal world and this sense of belonging constitutes a fundamental and unavoidable need. The chapter describes the best techniques to relate to these clients in group and prevent them from becoming scapegoats as a primitive defense during difficult and painful evolutionary moments.

Chapter 16 is dedicated to depressive and bipolar disorders through the detailed account of a clinical case. Group therapy is particularly suitable for clients suffering from mood disorders, since it facilitates compliance and stabilizes the alliance thanks to the diverse contribution of each member, who have the power not only to welcome but also to confront anger inhibition and support a healthy expression of repressed feelings in order to give a more constructive direction to the interpersonal life of those suffering from depression. When their suffering is characterized by dysthymia and instability, the group fosters acceptance of their biologic vulnerability and a prospective need to take up pharmacological treatment.

Chapter 17 tackles the complex process of the end of group therapy, the current criteria for a proper conclusion, and the changes the entire group must face when a member leaves the group at the end of their journey. Ending therapy as per agreement with therapist and group allows a sort of protection for the time immediately after. Clients leaving the group take with them valuable feedback that will guide them, in the years to come, to the end of their journey. They also enjoy the social recognition of having achieved awareness and control over their symptoms, and understand the depths of the personal changes with which they face separations. Experiencing a joyful and victorious separation is a resource for the future and, for some, a first instance of relational learning about the mourning process. All group members learn something in saying goodbye to a fellow member leaving in a positive manner and can gain invaluable insight even when someone interrupts treatment precociously. This chapter also explores the difficulties of therapy and its interruption.

Chapter 18 presents a group session. Group members participated in the writing of the chapter. It is difficult to represent theoretically what happens in a session: That is why we deemed it more useful to narrate a moment of therapy, with all the richness of interpersonal transactions which would provide enough material for a screenplay, instead of confining ourselves to a detailed analysis of the exchanges. People's thoughts, which they act on through their behaviors and words, are very intense and swift, and make for the type of material extremely rich in themes that are recognizable also for the repetitive traits of the script patterns. There is a sort of theatre in which everyone improvises, and the therapist observes, participates, and from time to time provides elements useful to alter the pattern and enrich the exchange.

While we were finishing this book, the world was overcome by the Covid-19 pandemic, forcing us to move our work online. For this reason, too, Chapter 19 is dedicated to the conduction of online groups and focuses on the most current studies on the efficacy of this type of therapy. The dimension of virtual relationships in the midst of a historic metamorphosis requires the courage to break new grounds and explore new modes of intervention, reconfiguring a setting while including a constructive adaptation of the technique used up until now and keeping in touch with our clients in a meaningful way. It is mostly a visual touch and it pushes us to practice in the recognition of emotions communicated through facial expressions and looks. This chapter reports the recent experience that allowed us to continue the therapeutic work remotely and witness first-hand the importance of learning from the here-and-now, adapting to new tools and bringing hope and communality in a difficult moment of forced isolation to spur often unexpected syntonizations.

Chapter 20 examines the benefits and limits of group therapy, therapists' training, and supervision. Each educational journey, beside a thorough theoretical exploration of a clinically useful model, should develop the therapeutic resources that each trainee already carries within themselves carried within the personality of each trainee and among these, the desire to learn, learn from experience, and learn to think without fear. The permission to think is at the basis of a psychotherapist's training. A psychotherapist-in-training who feels recognized by their class and teachers in the expression of their thoughts and ideas, who feels free to explore, ask questions, and put themselves to the test in the knowledges of doing and being, – through theoretical lessons, practical workshops, role-playing sessions, and traineeships – is able to develop complex abilities allowing them to integrate information coming from different sources: theories, personal affective relationships, clients' verbal, and non-verbal communication.

At the end of the book, we have attached an appendix in which we summarize the stages of development that characterize the structuring of an individual's personality according to transactional analysis, in order to facilitate comprehension of some complex ideas herein described (especially for those readers who are unfamiliar with the transactional analysis model).

1

WHY THE GROUP?

Alone together

The existential condition of being "alone together" is typical of this day and age. It is the condition of the Facebook user who, through a computer screen, finds themselves in touch with the world. The same can be said for the new political movements that are taking the streets: thanks to social networks like Twitter, it is easier to organize large gatherings of people, and it is just as easy for these gatherings to quickly disperse.

In her book *Alone Together: Why We Expect More From Technology and Less From Each Other* (2011), psychologist Sherry Turkle presents the results of an interesting clinical and ethnographical study on the relationship between individuals and technology, aiming at understanding how the web and the automation processes are changing our lives and shaping our identities. The author observed and interviewed more than 450 people: 300 young students belonging to different American schools and college campuses, and 150 adults. She found, for example, that the Internet and social networks make us "richer" in terms of acquaintances, yet these "friendships" are ever more precarious and short-lived. A number of other studies highlight how an average American in the age of Facebook, LinkedIn, and other social networks actually has fewer friends they meet in person compared to 10 or 20 years ago. We are giving up direct human contact in the name of technology, and a fear of disconnection is emerging, denominated by researchers as FOMO, *Fear of Missing Out* (Hunt, Marx, Lipson, & Young, 2018). We prefer to chat for hours through a profile or avatar often hiding our true face and name.

Technologies seem safer to us because virtual relationships are easier to manage and control, but most of all, they look like they are less subject to unforeseen turns of events. Digital culture gives us the illusion that we are all part of a community, whereas in reality, we are all more alone than ever. The consequences of this condition on our brain are still an object of study and research. The basis for Turkle's reasoning can be found in the idea of a "fragmented ego," and these ego fragments are distributed throughout the different virtual experiences and relationships with online contacts. According to the sociologist, the social and

DOI: 10.4324/9781003215547-2

psychological aspects of these virtual experiences and relationships actually contribute to build up the individual personalities of the subjects that are experiencing them, exactly as – symbolically speaking – the many windows that make up the graphic interface of every operative system. Additionally, Turkle believes that web-based communication will gradually help us to conceive human identity as more fluid and complete, and allow us to perceive the many different egos coexisting inside ourselves. In her essay *Life on the Screen* (1995), Turkle stresses again that in environments mediated by digital interfaces, the ego is indeed manifold, and it interacts with other users rather fluidly through those same digital interfaces. Thanks to this network, individuals can communicate across the board with a potentially endless number of people belonging to different geographical areas, genders, and cultures: in a virtual reality, for example, they can embody a different gender identity, and in doing so, they might be able to widen their knowledge of that gender much more than they had ever thought possible; they might also be inclined to express more freely certain intellectual attitudes or psychological dispositions which would have had a harder time surfacing outside of a virtual context. According to Turkle, the plurality of egos manifested online is not identifiable with a psychotic symptom: quite the contrary, digital reality, encouraging the creation and accessibility of virtual worlds, may constitute a balancing factor with regard to the complexity of each individual's personality. The required condition is that the individual in question manage to use the interactive experience offered by the web as a trampoline to acquire a certain set of competences and to increase emotional security also outside of virtual reality.

Building a social brain

If for years researchers have studied the brain as an element of its own, taking it out of its social context, today we know that it owes its survival to its interactions with others.

According to Alexander (1989), a well-known evolutionary biologist, our ancestors might have developed a complex brain in order to be able to negotiate and manage complex social interactions. A specific characteristic which sets apart human beings from other animal species is their capability to understand others' thought processes through empathy and self-awareness. Alexander believes that our intelligence did not evolve to fight adverse natural conditions but to be able to compete with other individuals of our same species: the ability to comprehend the mental states of others as well as our own, called mentalization,[1] evolved so as to allow us to surpass our equals in shrewdness and cleverness. Since *Homo sapiens* is a social creature, their ability to "read" the mind of their peers allow them to quickly identify the elements on which others focus their attention, and to speculate with regard to their intentions and evaluation of events. Moreover, their ability to recognize non-verbal cues helps to access hidden aspects of other people's minds, granting them a constructive influence on others.

9

Many neuropsychological studies today confirm that the development of the prefrontal cortex matches that of mentalization, of behavior prediction, and of emotional regulation processes. Thus, changes in brain structure are associated with the evolution of social intelligence: a slight proportioned expansion in the prefrontal cortex areas, around ten percent (Semendeferi & Damasio, 2000), was accompanied by an increase of neuronal interconnections in those areas. This expansion was also followed by an increase in volume of the right prefrontal cortex, an area involved in self-awareness, and the ability to remember personal experiences and plan for the future. According to Alexander, the right prefrontal cortex may help us find "a way of seeing ourselves as others see us so that we may cause competitive others to see us as we wish them to" (1990, p. 7).

Social interactions and mentalization

The role of mentalization, then, is not just to encourage collaboration and positive relationships, but most of all social survival. In a way, the ability to build healthy and authentic human relationships truly amounts to an evolutionary advantage. Environmental interactions, there since the very first stages of development, contribute to the "social building" of the brain: it is our ability to establish constructive relations with others that actually molds our brain.

Massimo Ammaniti in his interesting book *Noi. Perché due sono meglio di uno* (2014),[2] writes:

> Going back to child development, there is consistent proof that we look for interactions with others even from birth, if not before, and that there is a relentless need to understand codes of exchanges and social interactions.
> This specific disposition to sociality would represent a peculiarity of the human species which is absent in animals, since mutual aid may have significantly helped humans adapt and survive.
>
> (p. 11)[3]

> Anthropologist Robin Dunbar established a connection between size of the brain, mostly of the neocortex, and size of the groups in which the different species live. . . . A bigger group takes care of the individual, may be able to protect it from harsh environments and also contributes to the development of a more sophisticated brain structure.
>
> (p. 102)

"When we interact with others or think about others, there is an activation of the medial areas of the brain such as the cingulate gyrus or the medial prefrontal cortex" (Ammaniti, 2014, p. 103). Some psychobiologists (Lieberman, 2013) speculate on the existence of a *default mode network*, a neural network distributed in different subcortical regions which activates during rest hours. The cognitive skills involved in this mechanism are the ability to reflect on and evaluate one's own mental states and emotions as well as others': it is a cerebral system of social representation which works even when the mind is at rest. These aspects correspond to what Berne calls "group imago" (Berne, 1963). So, the *default system* works to regulate the relation between self and others and make it predictable and manageable: in fact, it remains running in the background even during sleep and dreams. Additionally, studies on the reward system (Shulman et al., 2016) confirm an interesting data: the ventral striatum – the region of the brain responsible for satisfaction – activates when we develop cooperative behaviors and we feel welcomed by the social group. On the other hand, the cingulate cortex is responsible for the great sufferance set off by experiences of exclusion, thus confirming that experiences of reciprocity are encouraged and supported by our brain. This principle also regulates human communication in what concerns sharing and reciprocity: when arriving at the office, we say "what a nice day" even just to share a feeling, and this kind of communication is fundamental in order to boost connections with others (Tomasello, 2009). The *we* is inside our brain, our emotional system, our language, and the more human we are, the more plural we become.

Brain plasticity and environmental enrichment

Recent neuroscientific studies explain how some experiences are crucial to brain plasticity. The concept of plasticity is related to that of vulnerability to environmental stimuli and, on its own, it is neither positive nor negative. However, if the stimuli are positive, there is space to learn, grow, and even fix former negative experiences. Neuroscientist Berardi writes:

> The plasticity of the brain shows that the brain is prepared to grow in a context characterized by safety, positive excitement, sincere shared availability and exploration. A large social group, the presence of several objects which stimulate curiosity, exploration and productive activities, the possibility to do voluntary physical exercise. What are the key-words when it comes to environmental enrichment? We have learned they are, of course, cognitive and physical activity, social interactions, novelties, but also interest, motivation, curiosity, satisfaction. Animals living in an enriched environment are not forced to do anything at all; if they run on the wheel we can infer that they are motivated to do so. Thus, an enriched environment is a possibility from which each subject extracts what gives them the most satisfaction. In adult animal specimens an "enriched" lifestyle leads to better performances in learning and memorization tasks (they learn faster and rarely forget) and to an increased behavioral flexibility. There is similar evidence for humans as well. How can enriched environments even have such effects? It is very simple: environmental enrichment affects all the known factors of synaptic plasticity.
>
> (2019, p. 45)

As we have seen and will continue to explore later, parental mirroring helps guiding children through a journey that begins with birth and leads them to become part of a social mind. When this mirroring fails, group therapy stands a chance to fix this failure: in-group is indeed possible to learn how to think instead of act, how to think about oneself and one's history, and how to build different narrations of oneself and others and to share these with the group. The social brain builds itself through relationships. In group, therapist and members are involved in a process that connects "left brain" and "right brain" (Hargaden & Sills, 2002), in which the group acts as a container, facilitating members' emotional regulation. Indeed, members often manage to experience their feelings only after having recognized them in another or through another. Group therapy then becomes an enriched environment, crucial to the activation of new reparative and formative synaptic processes.

Language, body, and studies on groups

In this book, we will discuss how an up-to-date transactional analysis should keep studying languages and emotional experiences that facilitate synaptic changes. Today, to explain what really happens with communication in a therapy setting and what is the role of the therapist in it, it is necessary to combine Berne's intuitions with the study of Wilma Bucci's multiple code theory (1997). Today's therapists should know how the different codes function, as well as to be able to describe the sub-symbolic level which dominates group interactions.

We will also discuss Schore's (2003) studies on the right brain and its correlations to therapeutic group work. Following Cornell's (2015) studies, we will then see how the group represents a profoundly corporeal experience and how this dimension remains even in an online setting.

We strongly believe that these integrations will promote a new transactional analysis that, in Berne's spirit, will follow the thrilling new research of this day and age in neuroscience and neuropsychoanalysis.

The group setting and the cognitive nature of therapeutic operations together with the regressive and oneiric atmosphere – the latter of which facilitates the expression of transference processes and a deep reorganization of the self – constitute a truly rich wealth of experiences for a relevant psychodynamic psychotherapy, one that nurtures intersubjectivity and the We. In a group setting, experiencing the "present moment," as Daniel Stern (2004) would say, aids the learning of new coping strategies and the emotional growth of each member. This is especially important today. In the world of the fourth revolution (Floridi, 2017), in which disconnection from digital information and social networks represents the first form of anxiety, group therapy may help many people find a new kind of balance between their online presence and their "unplugged" life between isolation and affective belonging, helping them develop an authentic sense of self along with a sense of belonging to a broader We.

Notes

1 The ability to draw inferences based on the internal states and intentions of others as well as our own (Bateman & Fonagy, 2006).
2 *[Us. Why two is better than one].* My translation.
3 My translation.

References

Alexander, R. D. (1989). Evolution of the human psyche. In C. Stringer & P. Mellars (Eds.), *The human revolution: Behavioral and biological perspectives on the origins of modern humans* (pp. 455–513). Princeton, NJ: Princeton University Press.

Alexander, R. D. (1990). *How did humans evolve? Reflections on the uniquely unique species.* Ann Arbor: University of Michigan, Museum of Zoology.

Ammaniti, M. (2014). *Noi: Perché due sono meglio di uno.* Bologna: Il Mulino.

Bateman, A., & Fonagy, P. (2006). *Mentalization-based treatment for borderline personality disorder: A practical guide.* Oxford: Oxford University Press. doi:10.1093/med/9780198570905.001.0001

Berardi, N. (2019). Cervello e comportamento. *Percorsi di Analisi Transazionale, IV*(3), 36–59.

Berne, E. (1963). *The structure and dynamics of organizations and groups.* New York: Grove Press.

Bucci, W. (1997). Symptoms and symbols: A multiple code theory of somatization. *Psychoanalytic Inquiry, 17*(2), 151–172. doi:10.1080/07351699709534117

Cornell, W. F. (2015). *Somatic experience in psychoanalysis and psychotherapy: In the expressive language of the living.* London: Routledge. Retrieved from www.taylorfrancis.com/books/e/9781317575399

Floridi, L. (2017). *La quarta rivoluzione: Come l'infosfera sta trasformando il mondo.* Milano: Raffaello Cortina.

Hargaden, H., & Sills, C. (2002). *Transactional analysis: A relational perspective.* New York: Brunner-Routledge.

Hunt, M. G., Marx, R., Lipson, C., & Young, J. (2018). No more FOMO: Limiting social media decreases loneliness and depression. *Journal of Social and Clinical Psychology, 37*(10), 751–768. doi:10.1521/jscp.2018.37.10.751

Lieberman, M. D. (2013). *Social: Why our brains are wired to connect.* New York: Crown Publishers.

Schore, A. N. (2003). *Affect regulation & the repair of the self.* New York: W.W. Norton.

Semendeferi, K., & Damasio, H. (2000). The brain and its main anatomical subdivisions in living hominoids using magnetic resonance imaging. *Journal of Human Evolution, 38*(2), 317–332. doi:10.1006/jhev.1999.0381

Shulman, E. P., Smith, A. R., Silva, K., Icenogle, G., Duell, N., Chein, J., & Steinberg, L. (2016). The dual systems model: Review, reappraisal, and reaffirmation. *Developmental Cognitive Neuroscience, 17*, 103–117. doi:10.1016/j.dcn.2015.12.010

Stern, D. N. (2004). *The present moment in psychotherapy and everyday life.* New York: W.W. Norton.

Tomasello, M., & Restani, D. (2009). *Altruisti nati: Perché cooperiamo fin da piccoli.* Torino: Bollati Boringhieri.

Turkle, S. (1995). *Life on the screen: Identity in the age of the Internet.* New York: Touchstone.

Turkle, S. (2011). *Alone together: Why we expect more from technology and less from each other.* New York: Basic Books.

2

GROUP THEORY

In this chapter, we will take a look at the history of group theory from Le Bon's (1896) and McDougall's (1920) first studies on the effect of groups on individuals, up until Freud's (1921) pioneering work on group psychology.

We will provide an overview of the authors who worked directly with psycho-analytical therapeutic groups, underlining the influence these had on more recent theories on group psychotherapy and most of all on the ideas we will discuss in this volume. We will look for points of contact between the work of these authors and transactional analysis methodology. We believe that it is useful to explore the theory of group therapy, since often psychotherapists come to this type of treatment from the experience acquired with individual psychotherapy. In group, how-ever, there is an intersection of individual and group dynamics, themes related to individuality and intimacy, and we feel it is only appropriate to consider both perspectives. Starting from group dynamics to then move on to individual ones allows us to take a broader look at group processes and avoids focalizing on the contents brought up by individual members. In this way, group theory offers an important contribution to understand group dynamics within the therapeutic process.

Le Bon (1896) and McDougall (1920) were among the first to study the psychology behind large groups of people and to describe the influence these had on the individual's behavior. Le Bon uses terms such as *contagion* and *hypnotic suggestion* to remark on the "primitive" nature of crowd behavior, pointing out that individuals, when they are part of a crowd, lose their identity and their sense of responsibility.

According to Le Bon, crowds in and of themselves tend to regression:

> By the mere fact that he forms part of an organized crowd, a man descends several rungs in the ladder of civilization. Isolated, he may be a cultivated individual; in a crowd, he is a barbarian – that is, a creature acting by instinct.
>
> (p. 8)

McDougall agrees with Le Bon about the degrading power the group has on individuals. However, he claims that the group might also be able to elevate

   DOI: 10.4324/9781003215547-3

individual behavior. According to McDougall, unorganized groups are in fact the ones to manifest impulsive and violent behavior, and are ruled by the power of the unconscious. However, he believes that an organized group, with shared and openly formulated goals, might facilitate the differentiation of each member's function and foster a constructive feeling of continuity, thus leaving behind uncontrolled regressive experiences and evolving to a superior level.

In *Group Psychology and The Analysis of The Ego* (1921), Freud, taking as a starting point the ideas developed by Le Bon and McDougall, analyzes the behavior exhibited by an individual interacting with a wider group of strangers. In opposition to the two sociologists, Freud claims that what keeps individuals together is not the hypnotic suggestion but the libidinal ties developed between group members, as well as between these and the leader.

Taking as an example organized collectivities such as the army or the church, he suggests that what keeps member together is the illusion that everyone is loved equally by the supreme leader. The common habit of overestimation and idealization of the leader would cause within each individual a regression and an undifferentiation, thus inhibiting their capacity to think autonomously.

Group theory in practice

The first pioneering attempt to organize a group psychotherapy session is attributed to Joseph Pratt, an internal medicine physician at Boston's Massachusetts General Hospital (Pratt, 1969). In 1905, Pratt brought together a group of 15 patients affected by tuberculosis with the aim to make them discuss their common problems and learn from each other. Pratt reported very positive results from this new type of treatment. The patients' morale improved significantly thanks to the group's supportive atmosphere. The method he followed may be compared to today's psychoeducational model.

The application of group therapy to the psychotherapeutic context dates back to Edwards Lazell, who, in 1919, at St. Elisabeths's Hospital in Washington, started treating psychiatric patients, especially those suffering from schizophrenia, using a "talk therapy" (Lazell, 1921). His method consisted in inviting patients for whom individual psychotherapy had been ineffective to take part in a series of conferences centered around the emotional aspects of their pathology. Each conference was followed by a moment of sharing between psychiatrist and patients. Lazell observed that, during this particular moment, patients left their usual state of dullness and withdrawal and "came to life again," actively participating in the interactions.

Trigant Burrow is credited by many authors (Migone, 1995) with having coined the term *group analysis*. Burrow (1927) claimed the existence of a "natural interfunctioning" between human beings, anticipating by many years the studies related to this topic. According to this author, whose thought shares some similarities with Berne's, social dynamics are at the basis of both personality development and mental disorders. Thus, the latter may be better analyzed within a group setting. It is worth noting, at this point, that Berne considered TA as a branch of social psychiatry, of which group psychotherapy represented the preferred site of observation and treatment (Berne, 1966). Burrow, much like Berne, was unsatisfied by the importance that psychoanalysis attributed to individuals, who, according to the author, could not be considered without taking into account their social environment. He was convinced that in a group setting, clients might be able to develop an awareness of their distorted self-image through discussing it openly with others.

The therapist was supposed to join the other members in the exploration of the reciprocal unconscious dynamics emerging in the here-and-now of the group process. As William Cornell wrote: "He argued that in group analytic work, the analyst could not hold a privileged position. . . . Everyone in the group was an observer of his or her own processes and was observed and analyzed by everyone else" (Cornell, De Graaf, Newton, & Thunnissem, 2016, p. 138).

His was an experiential study, conducted with his collaborators, students, and clients with whom he went to live on the Adirondack Mountains, in the state of New York. This type of setting preceded the "new groups" developed in California from the 1960s with the spread of group marathons, meditation, and sensory awareness groups, etc. Because of his research into group psychoanalysis, Burrow was spurned by the *American Psychoanalytic Association* in 1933. This open conflict with classic psychoanalytical tradition is another point of contact between Burrow and Berne: the latter, as remarked by Filanti and Attanasio Romanini (2017), claimed that Burrow was the only American psychiatrist to have developed interesting ideas on group therapy. Berne was saddened by the fact that Burrow's studies on groups had been basically ignored because of his unorthodox positions and he insisted "he may be regarded as the outstanding pioneer in the whole science of the study of small groups" (Berne, 1963, p. 289).

In their book *Psychoanalysis in Groups* (1962), Wolf and Schwartz described a method called "group psychoanalysis" which consisted in the use, within the context of group therapy, of analytical instruments such as free association, transference, and dream analysis. According to this perspective, each group member undergoes a one-on-one session with the therapist at the same time as the others: thus, the therapist works with each client without taking into consideration members' interactions. This approach will also be put into practice in a transactional analysis context by the Gouldings (Goulding & Goulding, 1979).

Experiential groups

Kurt Lewin (1951), an important representative of Gestalt psychology, influenced by Planck's studies on force fields in physics, applied the concept of *force field* to personality development. He postulated the existence of a state of balance between the individual and its environment. The upsetting of this balance gives way to a tension which, in turn, provokes an alteration aiming to restore it. Within the group-field, each individual influences other people and the group itself with their actions, thus creating some sort of interdependence between each member and the group, as well as between members themselves.

According to Lewin, the resultant of the forces that act on the individual and the group is not to be found in members' past lives but in the here-and-now. These forces can be identified as group's goals, cohesion, roles, leadership style, etc. T-groups (also known as *sensitive training groups*) were born in 1945 in the United States, when Lewin, who was working at MIT at the time, found that feedback given to members with regard to their attitudes and modes of interactions was an effective therapeutic factor from both a cognitive and an emotional point of view, encouraging changes at a personal, social, and organizational level. After his death in 1947, his students kept practicing group therapy in Bethel, Maine.

Parallel to Lewin's work, at the University of Chicago, Carl Rogers (1970) developed an approach to the conduction of small groups that was aimed at personal growth and the improvement of interpersonal relationships. Rogerian groups are characterized by a more experiential and therapeutic approach if compared to Lewin's, which mostly focused on improving efficacy and the group climate. On this matter, Rogers declared: "The Chicago groups were oriented primarily toward personal growth and the development and improvement of interpersonal communication and relationships, rather than having these as secondary aims . . . than the groups originating in Bethel" (Rogers, 1970, p. 4).

The group as a whole

Bion's *Experiences in Groups* (1959) is still considered relevant and meaningful in the landscape of psychoanalytical group psychology. It is an essay collection inspired by the real-life experiences of the author, who, during World War II, served as a psychiatrist in a military hospital in England, as Berne himself did. The book also takes its cue from another one of Bion's experiences, this time at Tavistock Clinic in London, of which he was an important member. About him, Berne would say: "Bion has studied carefully certain important aspects of group psychology and has re-emphasized the value of observing groups in a naturalistic and unprejudiced way" (Berne, 1963, p. 288).

Bion does not see the group simply as individuals gathered together, but as a whole entity, in which he distinguishes two layers: A manifest layer focused on the task and the aim, which he defines as *work group*, and a hidden layer, based on anxieties and primitive fears, which is constituted by *basic assumptions*. The latter are unconscious, but they still have a great influence in the group process.

Bion postulates the existence of three types of basic assumptions:

1   *Basic assumption of dependence*: The group's belief that the leader might be able to satisfy everybody's needs, which makes it so that there are numerous expectations projected onto the therapist. If the latter is unable to identify this assumption, the group runs the risk of becoming dependent from the leader, thus giving up its autonomy.

2   *Basic assumption of fight-flight*: The group's belief that there is an outside
    enemy that they need to attack or from whom they need to flee. When the
    group develops this defensive split perhaps one or more members risk being
    relegated into the role of scapegoat (Cornell et al., 2016).
3   *Basic assumption of pairing*: The group's messianic hope that needs that gen-
    erate intense negative emotions will be satisfied by a yet unborn being. This
    assumption is often developed around the end of treatment to avoid the pain
    of separation. In order for this basic assumption to remain, it is important that
    the group's aim is never achieved so that a constant tension toward something
    can be maintained.

According to Bion, therapists have the responsibility to help group members
understand the expressions of basic assumptions in order to free themselves from
dependence and enter into a satisfying equal relationship with other members.
This methodology is still practiced today by therapists who use a transactional
analysis approach. Additionally, it is particularly useful with regard to organizational and training groups. In fact, basic assumptions can also be found in these
types of groups, and only through the recognition and elaboration of these regressive drives, it is possible to facilitate the development of collaborative dynamics
between members.

The group is considered as a whole in Adrienne Lee's (2014) model as well. In
it, clients are guided by the leader through the elaboration of the archaic themes
that emerge during group process. The aim is to enjoy new, open, and flexible
experiences in the here-and-now, and meaningful affective relational models. In
Bion's words, we could define this aim as the transformation of a group running
on basic assumptions into a work group.

A contemporary of the force field theory developed by Lewin in the United
States is group analysis, developed by Foulkes in England: a form of psychotherapy "*by* the group, *of* the group, including its conductor" (Foulkes, 1975, p. 3).

Profoundly influenced by classic Gestalt psychology, Foulkes, too, claims that
the group is more than the sum of its parts and that no individual can be analyzed
outside of its social context. His theory is based on the idea of a web of communication which creates a "group matrix." This matrix, in turn, develops and takes
on different traits and characteristics following the evolution of the group process.
According to Foulkes, the therapist's task is to widen and deepen communication
in order to facilitate comparisons between group members, a phenomenon he calls
"mirror reaction." Today, the latter is still considered to be a powerful therapeutic
factor also in transactional analysis, offering a chance at integration to all kinds of
clients. It is particularly useful for clients suffering from narcissistic personality
disorder, who were precluded, at an early age, the possibility to see themselves
reflected in the caregiver's role. Additionally, Berne greatly appreciates Foulkes's
attempt – which he considers successful – to draw its concepts from the direct
observation of group dynamics, instead of borrowing them from individual psychotherapy (Berne, 1963).

Among the authors Berne often references in his works related to group psychotherapy, beside Burrow, Bion, and Foulkes, we find Henry Ezriel, a psychoanalyst who participated in Bion's first group but ended up distancing himself from it shortly after, favoring Melanie Klein's object relation theory over Bion's model.

Ezriel (1973) introduces the concept – of Lewinian origins – of a "common group tension," to describe the group conflict arising from three different types of transference: required transference, avoided transference, and calamity. The "required" transference is the relationship the client establishes with the therapist in order to "avoid" the "calamity." In order to provide an exhaustive interpretation, the therapist has to refer to all three types of transference and show each member what their own personal contribution to the conflict and its resolution is. Suppose, for example, that members were discussing how the group may touch on many intellectual topics but actually lacks any real emotional sharing. Ezriel, focusing on the way each member expresses personal conflict, may speculate that the group is here referring to an excess of analysis and a lack of spontaneity (required relationship) in order to avoid criticizing the therapist (avoided relationship) and mostly to avoid being rejected by the therapist (calamity). Although he remained secondary to Bion, the fact that Ezriel put on the same level the group as a whole and members' individual experiences, and focused on transference in the here-and-now, makes his theory still rather relevant. Berne especially appreciates the implication of Ezriel's observations that what happens within the group is essentially based on transference (Berne, 1963).

According to Whitaker and Lieberman's (1964) focal conflict theory, the group is conceived as a whole and it is the privileged object of the therapist's attention, who, however, directs his interpretations also to the individual members. The aim of this model is the integration of Lewin's work with psychoanalytic practice. Whitaker and Lieberman believe that all clients' behaviors during a session may be interpreted as attempts to avoid a conflict within the group between a "disturbing motive," made of a desire or a need, and a "reactive" motive, that is, a fear associated with the gratification of said desire. This theory postulates that the group is constantly and unwittingly engaged in this conflict and it is always looking for a compromise in order to fulfill its desire and reduce anxieties associated with reactive fear. The disturbing motives can be of various nature: an aggressive attitude toward the therapist, a desire to be the center of attention, and sexual drives. To these disturbing motives correspond just as much reactive motives: fear of offending the therapist, fear of abandonment, fear of criticism, fear of annihilation, and fear of losing control of one's own sexual and aggressive emotions. After having processed and clarified these conflicts, the group can enter a new stage free of anxieties, during which a deeper and more intimate matter can emerge among members. The therapist's correct interpretations identify the focal conflict, thus facilitating a sense of safety within the group, "a progressive group culture," as Whitaker and Lieberman define it, offering clients a space where they can understand and leave behind recurring maladaptive behaviors. According to Hargaden and Sills (2002), focal conflict theory allows us to understand very well what happens when the group finds itself facing difficult situations. To be exact, only if each member takes the others' conflicts as their own, the group will be able to grow and its members will be able to acknowledge and integrate their split parts. If a conflict remains unprocessed, because, for example, as it is often the case, the therapist fails to analyze their own countertransference; it might cause the person who generated the conflict to leave the group or to be excluded by others, thus blocking the growth and development of the group itself.

Approaching interpersonal learning

Yalom and Leszcz (2005) follow the interpersonal theory formulated by Henry Sullivan, an American psychiatrist who shares several similarities with Berne. Sullivan, too, like Berne, regards interpersonal relations as incredibly important for the development of the individual's personality. Yalom does not exclude the concept of the group as a whole but considers it of a minor importance, mostly focusing on interpersonal interactions and transactions within the group setting. According to Yalom, in fact, change happens in the here-and-now group interactions through feedbacks and self-observation (Yalom & Leszcz, 2005; Rutan & Alonso, 1982). As we will explore later, his technique is very close to that of transactional analysis. Through the experiences that happen within the group setting, clients become aware of their own maladaptive interpersonal interactions and distorted perceptions, which may cause other members' negative or undesirable reactions. During this process, what takes place is a "corrective emotional experience" which mostly happens when we take into consideration human interactions in the here-and-now.

References to TA literature on groups and conclusions

The authors we have herein mentioned belong to the psychoanalytical world but, as Cornell (2020) reminds us, Berne, in his book *Principles of Group Treatment* (1966), kept his psychodynamic roots by referring to at least 25 authors belonging to the psychoanalytic current.

We have seen how a focus on the inner life of the individual (the intrapsychic component), on the relational styles (the interpersonal component), and on the group's social structure (the sociopsychological component) constitutes the foundation of all the different perspectives of psychodynamic psychotherapy.

We have observed three different approaches: the first, in which the group is used as a setting for individual therapy, while everyone else acts as a sounding board in which unconscious emotions can vibrate and resonate; the second, in which the group as a whole becomes object of treatment and the therapist relates to it as if it were an individual; finally, the most widely used today, the interpersonal learning approach, which focuses on group interactions in the here-and-now.

Eric Berne describes our therapy method as a group therapy method. He presented it this way to the scientific community in his first articles (1958) and then in *Transactional Analysis in Psychotherapy*, published in 1961.

We know that, after Berne, the 1970s led to divisions within TA and a multiplication of techniques and types of group setting. Those who opted to integrate TA with Gestalt psychology chose group marathons as a setting and redecision therapy (Goulding) as a technique. Within the therapeutic community, Schiff's model (Schiff, 1975) used a transactional analysis setting in order to undertake psychoeducational work with clients who suffered from severe psychotic and borderline disorders and had previous experiences of drugs and alcohol addiction.

Those who opted to keep following the classic Bernian method favored a weekly group setting of an hour and a half or two hours, in which the cognitive transactional aspects had the most relevance compared to other techniques and methodologies. Thus, in the classic group, they analyzed transactions and games; they used the whiteboard and experimented with ways of changing the stroke system and improving emotional and relational skills. This model led to two meaningful evolutions in the 1990s, namely integrative TA and psychodynamic TA. The former highlights the empathetic impact of the group as main therapeutic factor. The latter, building on Berne's psychoanalytic roots, focuses on the interpretative techniques of group transference. Here, each client's group imago is seen and analyzed as a projective experience, thus revealing the script they enact within their relationships.

The psychodynamic TA model, enriched by relational-TA-based ideas and by the now widespread experience of relational psychoanalysis, represents the main focus of our clinical practice.

We consider its group setting particularly useful to do deconfusion work – the deepest work on the client's psyche in TA – because we believe that it is the most powerful and potentially transformative for clients, especially if compared to individual therapy. The latter involves, from our perspective, a greater risk of keeping clients in regressive symbiotic relationships, that is, in a pathological condition.

In the 2013 debate published on the *Transactional Analysis Journal* monographic issue dedicated to groups, Richard Erskine and William Cornell discussed thoroughly the relationship between a group therapy model based on recognitions and empathy (Erskine) and one centered on experiences of shame and confrontational techniques, the latter of which were more coherent with the Bernian methodology of treatment (Cornell). According to the latter, it is only within the group that members first get to re-experience and reenact their script beliefs, uncomfortable and painful feelings included, in order to find new ways to shape their relationship to the world.

Despite considering warmth and empathy to be a necessary underlining condition to therapy, we certainly find ourselves to be more in line with William Cornell's approach. Indeed, warmth and affection can only go so far: What really works as a treatment is the relearning experience. Thus, it is by practicing syntonization and dealing with relational break-ups that the clients will learn to be resilient and fix both other's and their own narcissistic wounds. Only this way is it possible to heal, that is, grow, mature, and learn how to be comfortable in our everyday life, expanding our options on how to live and what meaning to give to our existence into the world. For the very same reason, we deem useful the study of training groups, since they share with therapy groups a push toward members' individualization-differentiation, health, and autonomy, or, as we say today, toward the integrating Adult's power as the main ego state.

Indeed, Trudy Newton, an excellent researcher studying adults' training processes and TA professionals' training, states:

> Whenever we enter a new group – whether at work, socially, or for learning – we do so with an internal image or picture of how it will be and what our place will be in it. We are not usually aware that we do this, or that our picture is based on our experience of previous groups of which we have been part, right back to our primary group in the family. To start with, we will have places in our imago for the group leader and ourselves, and other people become differentiated as the group moves on, hopefully toward openness and autonomy. At first we may "see" only a few people as individuals, probably those who interact with us in ways that seem familiar. In a mature group, we will have a clear picture of each member and our relationship to him or her.
>
> (2003, p. 322)

De Graaf and Levy expand on this, saying:

> In our work as TA trainers, we feel the constant challenge to develop and maintain a learning climate in our training groups that is as safe as it can be and as disturbing as it should be.
>
> (2016, p. 230)

These considerations suggest that even in training groups, there lays a great opportunity of learning, since within the group itself, it is possible for all members to have concrete experiences of listening, communicating, negotiating, influencing each other, and improving their self-confidence through others' recognition. In group, it thus becomes possible to co-create new paths and give life new meanings.

References

Berne, E. (1958). Transactional analysis: A new and effective method of group therapy. *American Journal of Psychotherapy*, *12*(4), 735–743.

Berne, E. (1963/1973). *The structure and dynamics of organizations and groups*. New York: Ballantine.

Berne, E. (1966). *Principles of group treatment*. New York: Grove Press.

Bion, W. (1959). *Experiences in groups*. New York: Basic Books.

Burrow, T. (1927). The group method of analysis. *The Psychoanalytic Review*, *14*(268).

Cornell, W. F. (2020). Transactional analysis and psychoanalysis: Overcoming the narcissism of small differences in the shadow of Eric Berne. *Transactional Analysis Journal*, 164–178.

Cornell, W. F., De Graaf, A., Newton, T., & Thunnissem, M. (2016). *Into TA: A comprehensive textbook on transactional analysis*. London: Karnac Books Ltd.

De Graaf, A., & Levy, J. (2016). Are transactional analysis training program groups sufficiently disturbing? *Transactional Analysis Journal*, *46*(3), 222–231. doi:10.1177/0362153716648977

Ezriel, H. (1973). Psychoanalytic group therapy. In L. Wolberg (Eds.), *Group therapy* (pp. 183–210). New York: Stratton Intercontinental Medical Book.

Filanti, S., & Romanini Attanasio, S. (2017). *Il modello dell'Analisi Transazionale: Dai fondamenti teorici all'intervento*. Milano: Franco Angeli.

Foulkes, S. H. (1975). *Group analytic psychotherapy: Methods and principles*. London: Gordon & Breach.

Freud, S. (1921/2012). *Group psychology and the analysis of the ego*. Greensboro, NC: Empire Books.

Goulding, M., & Goulding, R. (1979). *Changing lives through redecision therapy*. New York: Brunner, Mazel.

Hargaden, H., & Sills, C. (2002). *Transactional analysis: A relational perspective*. New York: Brunner-Routledge.

Lazell, E. (1921). The group treatment of dementia praecox. *Psychoanalysis Revue*, *8*, 198.

Le Bon, G. (1896/2001). *The crowd: A study of the popular mind*. New York: Dover Publications.

Lee, A. (2014). The development of a process group. *Transactional Analysis Journal*, *44*, 41–52.

Lewin, K. (1951). *Field theory in social science: Selected theoretical papers*. New York: Harpers.

McDougall, W. (1920). *The group mind*. New York: G. P. Putnam's Sons.

Migone, P. (1995). Le Origini della Gruppoanalisi: Una Nota su Trigant Burrow. *Rivista Sperimentale di Freniatria*, *3*(CXIX), 512–517.

Newton, T. (2003). Identifying educational philosophy and practice through imagoes in transactional analysis training groups. *Transactional Analysis Journal*, *33*(4), 321331. doi:10.1177/036215370303300407

Pratt, J. (1969). The home sanatorium treatment of consumption. In H. Ruitembeek (Ed.), *Group therapy today*. New York: Atherton Press.

Rogers, C. (1970). *Carl Rogers on encounter groups*. New York: Harper & Row.

Rutan, J., & Alonso, A. (1982). Group therapy, individual or both? *International Journal of Group Psychotherapy*, *32*, 267–282.

Schiff, J. L. (1975). *Cathexis reader: Transactional analysis: Treatment of psychosis*. New York: Harper & Row.

Whitaker, D., & Lieberman, M. (1964). *Psychotherapy through the group process*. New York: Atherton Press.

Wolf, A., & Schwartz, E. (1962). *Psychoanalysis in groups*. New York: Grune & Stratton.

Yalom, I. D., & Leszcz, M. (2005). *The theory and practice of group psychotherapy* (5th ed.). New York: Basic Books (Originally published in 1970).

3

CHANGE AND EMPOWERMENT FACTORS IN GROUP

Therapy as a dance school

We have already mentioned how all of us are born from a "we" and only later become an "I." Indeed, we were born within a mother's body, so our heart started beating to the same rhythmic frequency as another heart: from the very beginning, we were always plural, intersubjective beings, and interconnected in a chemical and corporeal way to another being. Being born means, of course, separating and detaching oneself, but within us, the memory of the two hearts beating to the same rhythm lives on, and to grow means to experience the world walking on our own two legs, while at the same time perpetually looking for that lost original harmony.

Thus, in our journey, we begin from a "we," which then becomes an "I," which in turn goes finally back to the "we" of the couple, the group, the human community that is always, always plural. Paolo Apolito's (2014) wonderful book explained how our search for human contact goes back to the body's biological roots. We are driven by a biological impulse to move toward other people, to talk, to sing, to party, and to embrace. It is our nature that leads us to acknowledge each other through rhythm and music, language, and movement. There is neither merit nor choice in all this. We would all be happily open towards each other were it not for certain obstacles interfering, obstacles that we ourselves have historically created to divide us and wage war on each other.

The dialogue which stems from psychotherapy is akin to that between mother and child or between two lovers: it creates a synchronized rhythm and leads to our well-being, even beyond conscious processes and conversation topics.

On this matter, Tangolo writes:

> In my work as a therapist, I have always been struck by people who, since the first few sessions, seemed physically awkward, and had a hard time syntonizing their looks, their posture, their voice. These are people who interrupt you while you are speaking or cannot listen properly, and they always look like they are speaking to themselves. When they talk about unhappy relationships and feeling misunderstood by their family or colleagues, when they say they don't understand other people's

DOI: 10.4324/9781003215547-4

communication cues, what I hear is them expressing a real, deep struggle in interacting with others, in influencing their behaviors and in attracting affectionate and loving attentions. These people's misery is apparent during the session: they are dissonant, out of tune, and I do believe that only proper group therapy may be able to re-create that uterus from which to begin feeling once again in tune with others. . . . In such cases, I ask clients if they have had any experiences with swimming, dancing or caring for pets, if they sing or play a musical instrument in a band, if they have satisfying sexual encounters, and if they truly feel understood by someone during a conversation. Usually, the answer to all of these questions is that they feel awkward and out of tune with others during all these occasions of social pleasure. If they are at the center of attention, they may appear as either highly unpleasant or terribly alone, as narcissists in front of a mirror, closed off to any kind of contact, which, in the end, is really the true pleasure we find in sharing. Even in laughter people can be in or out of tune, and the pleasure of laughing together is similar to that of a chorus, an orgiastic dance, or a truly syntonized orgasm. During open-air folk festivals in Brittany and Ireland, I experienced folk dances which could last several hours. The Breton rhythms are ancient, and people take each other by the hand or even just by their little finger and let themselves be led away in dancing spirals and circles that go on and on in a hypnotic fashion until everyone is moving as one in unspeakable joy. . . . These are amongst the most satisfying experiences of my life because within rhythm and music our body and soul are one with others. . . . As Yalom (2001) brilliantly says, psychotherapy, too, must be a dance . . . and music school, a refined school of socialization which helps removing obstacles, rigidity, and blockages in syntonization, and encourages us to fill those empty places, those deficits that prevent each of us from being fully human: a body which feels all kinds of emotions, a soul attuned to the world and a mind that is always learning, every single day of our lives.

(Tangolo & Massi, 2015, p. 67)

Yalom's work

Irvin D. Yalom is considered the most influential scholar with regard to the research on the group's therapeutic factors. His handbook *The Theory and Practice of Group Psychotherapy* (Yalom & Leszcz, 2005) was included by *The American Journal of Psychiatry* among the ten most important psychiatry books published in the last few years.

To find the change factors operating within the group, Yalom used a tool called Q-sort: a list of 60 statements identifying 12 therapeutic factors, among which group members can indicate which are more helpful from their point of view. TA groups share several features with the therapeutic factors detected by Yalom.

We tried analyzing some of these therapeutic factors associating them with the main features of TA therapy groups. Finally, we selected a statement that exemplifies which new beliefs each factor contributes to create in clients about themselves, others, and life:

1   *Altruism*: Through their time with the group, members experience their own expertise and ability in satisfying other people's requests, without being relegated to the role of someone who needs help. In many of them, who often felt that they were a burden to others, the discovery of being important to someone else bolsters self-esteem, strengthens the Adult consciousness, and develops the Nurturing Parent. This is an important therapeutic factor to which clients undergoing individual therapy don't have access. The new reassessed beliefs this factor may contribute to create can be summarized in the following statement: *Helping others allows me to feel important, helps me to get out of the role of the helpless victim.*

2   *Interpersonal learning*: Through relationships with the therapist and other group members, clients learn that their maladaptive interpersonal interactions are often a product of the way they redefine others based on their own scripts, and sometimes these interactions give rise to negative or undesirable reactions from other members. The implicit mechanisms facilitating this learning process are not so much related to the interpretation or insight, as to the meaningful relational experiences lived in the here-and-now, and, in particular, to self-observation and feedback. For clients, group psychotherapy represents a corrective emotional experience (Alexander & French, 1946). They might access it exposing themselves, in favorable conditions, to emotional situations they have been incapable of facing in the past. The script beliefs that could previously be summarized into the statement *others don't see me or if they see me they criticize me*, now change into *understanding the others' impression of me helps me to become aware of my own behaviors, and offers me the possibility to change those behaviors that prevent others from understanding me.*

3   *Corrective recapitulation of the primary family group*: Clients who undertake group therapy have often had negative experiences with their family of origin. The group, in many ways similar to a family, enacts old family drama through a delicate interplay of transference and countertransference. With the help of the therapist and other members, this drama can be revisited and challenged (corrective emotional experience) in order to consider new behavioral models. Using a TA expression, we could say that the group allows clients to re-experience the script decisions of their childhood, to see them under a new light and become aware of new options. In this case, the new options can be summarized into the following statement: *Understanding the unfinished business in my old family relations allows me to face relationships with new groups from a more aware and determined point of view.*

27

4   *The instillation of hope*: Cheering each other up stimulates optimism between members and strengthens the feeling of being able to do it. The group is a source of strokes and support, both during and in between sessions. In particular, when group members develop a greater awareness and control on their games and resources, they also improve the quality of their social life, and in doing so, they earn from other members a supplementary dose of strokes, which will be helpful in strengthening their change process. Thanks to this therapeutic factor, the old script beliefs about themselves and *others* (*I'll never change, I'll never achieve the success I deserve*) will change into: *Being part of a group in which people improve encourages me to believe in myself and truly commit to change.*

5   *Development of socializing techniques*: Group therapy is very useful in understanding the social behavior each member exhibits often unwittingly. In particular, clients suffering from personality disorders tend to act out their interpersonal struggles and cannot put them into words. In direct contrast to one-on-one therapy, in group therapy, the enactments are immediately made apparent and dealt with. Through members' feedback, each client can become aware of their own maladaptive modes of social interactions, and, subsequently, learn new ones, thus considerably improving their social skills: This possibility represents a truly fundamental therapeutic factor. In TA, there are different therapeutic tactics and strategies selected depending on the type of client. The new beliefs generated by this therapeutic factor may be summarized in these statements: *Learning new modes of socialization gives me the opportunity to get closer to others* or *intimacy doesn't scare me anymore.*

6   *Imitative behaviors*: Clients have the possibility to observe and model themselves after the positive aspects of the therapist and other members' behaviors. For example, they might look at the way others deal with their problems, or at their availability to help other people. Imitative behavior may be assimilated to the twinning transference, one of Hargaden and Sills's (2002) introjective transferences. As all types of transference, it can foster development, thus allowing clients to experiment with new models of behavior. However, it may also engender defensive behaviors, leading the client to passively adapt to the behavioral models exhibited by the therapist and other members. It is the therapist's responsibility to differentiate these two modes of transference: this will help clients creatively synthetize the aspects of others they introject in order to form their own specific personality. Each member can choose one or more people to model themselves after in order to *try to be like somebody who is able to express themselves better than me.*

7   *Universality*: The "welcome to the human race" experience (Yalom & Leszcz, 2005) of those who come into the group is comprised of the revelation that other members have similar thoughts to their own, and it is deeply comforting. It allows the newcomer to escape their loneliness and more firmly develop their own sense of self. The fact that they are not alone in producing

28

thoughts that are generally abhorred by society allows the client to change their inner dialogue: where before the Critical Parent prevailed, now it is the Nurturing Parent to have the upper hand, and, subsequently, the Free Child to be more energized. *Sharing my problems with others makes me feel less alone* might become the client's new belief.

8   *Information*: The group fosters a sort of learning with regard to psychic functioning, symptoms' meanings, relational dynamics, and the therapeutic process. This therapeutic factor is also used in individual therapy: the difference, here, is that it is not just the therapist that gives information, but also members. In TA group therapy, knowing the Bernian theory, understanding what happens in various stages of the therapeutic journey and why, may help clients in developing a sense of mastery of the therapeutic experience and encourage cooperation in group work. In this setting, the awareness of the relational process is not just exclusive to the therapist, but it is extended to all members, thus facilitating the process of learning and promoting autonomy. Through this therapeutic factor, clients develop the new belief that *learning to get to know oneself and to understand the causes behind counterproductive behaviors aids the development of new, more functional, and adaptive skills.*

9   *Catharsis*: This factor is tied to the possibility of expressing openly and honestly one's most intimate feelings within a group. This is functional to the cohesion of the group, and, at the same time, it fosters in members an ability to deal with life's problems. Studies in oncological medicine, for example, tell us that being able to express in group therapy emotions related to an ill-omened diagnosis helps oncology patients overcome their feelings of helplessness and hopelessness, empowers them to acquire more responsibility in the therapeutic journey, and renders them more responsive to medical treatments (Fawzy & Fawzy, 1998). The client's new belief is that *the possibility to express real feelings, either positive or negative, without being judged for it* generates a better sense of self-efficacy and freedom to be themselves.

10 *Existential factors*: These factors were added later by Yalom and are related to the ability to access and accept fundamental aspects of our existence, such as death, the inevitability of loneliness, and taking responsibility for our own life. These factors, from a transactional analysis point of view, are functional to the decontamination of the Adult. *Taking responsibility for my choices means facing moments of deep loneliness; Life doesn't always offer me what I want and yet, it's still worth living; Dealing with painful moments allows me to be more detached when it comes to minor inconveniences*: These are the statements that express the new beliefs developed by clients in this case.

11 *Group cohesiveness*: This does not constitute a therapeutic factor in and of itself, but it is still an underlying condition that allows the development and efficacy of other factors. It represents the equivalent of building a solid "relationship" in individual therapy. Showing a better understanding and mutual acceptance, members of a cohesive group create an environment apt to self-expression and self-exploration, and, subsequently, develop a better

degree of self-awareness and personal growth. Group cohesion corresponds to the phase of the operative group imago (Berne, 1963), also called *norming* (Tuckman, 1965; Tuckman & Jensen, 1977). This is the phase of games and it registers an increased tolerance toward games and rackets. Members feel more secure within the group; they are more intuitive; and they communicate their emotions openly in a climate of mutual support. In a cohesive group, each member leaves behind the Don't Belong injunction, typical of the first few sessions, and instead grows to feel more *at home* inside the group.

Conclusions

The factors that help clients function better in a group generate a climate favorable to therapy: in and of itself, they are not enough to produce personal growth and change in the deep structures of personality, but they are essential like oxygen. To grow, we need food, water, strokes, and stimuli, but without oxygen life would not be possible.

Thus, it is necessary to complete these considerations on change factors with an analysis of setting conditions and basic group therapy techniques, without ever forgetting that the processes generating growth, healing from trauma, and deficit compensation are relational processes.

On this matter, Anna Massi writes:

> I believe this compensation to be facilitated within a psychotherapeutic group in which the profound sense of helplessness and isolation dissolves through the empathic, authentic encounter with others. Only where clients perceive a solid, trustworthy space, they will be able to turn their attention to their inner world, aware that that world does not possess the power to destroy anybody: not the therapist, not the group, and not themselves.
>
> (Tangolo & Massi, 2015, p. 80)

Later, she adds, with Anna Emanuela Tangolo:

> A person's growth goes through periods of intense emotion, crises, regressions and transformations; what happens within the individual also happens in group and one-on-one psychotherapy. In these circumstances, the therapeutic relationship repeats the clients' past failures so as to reframe them in a cooperative context and give them new meanings. For all our efforts, though, clients will never feel completely safe, and it is precisely this impossibility which will give way to change. The relations client/therapist, client/group are not a tool to free oneself from evolutionary trauma, as if the past was some kind of sickness, but a way to experience all together the meaning trauma brings with it, thus facilitating the emergence of the clients' natural ability to feel secure and joyful in their

nearness to others, as well as a durable stability of the self. The ability to take pleasure in our nearness to others is a natural talent but it is also a consequence of the development of the self. We are born. We grow. We develop. And during this development we are exposed to relational trauma, which inexorably reduces, through dissociation, our ability to place our full trust in our nearness to others. As Schore (2009) reminds us, nearness between an "I" and a "you" is a conversation between limbic systems, but, in order to fully explain this idea, we can consider the lyrics of the popular song The Nearness of You: It isn't your sweet conversation/ That brings this sensation/ Oh no, it's just the nearness of you.

(Tangolo & Massi, 2015, p. 80)

References

Alexander, F., & French, T. M. (1946). *Psychoanalytic therapy; principles and application*. New York: Ronald Press.

Apolito, P. (2014). *Ritmi di festa: Corpo, danza, socialità*. Bologna: Il Mulino.

Berne, E. (1963). *The structure and dynamics of organizations and groups*. New York: Grove Press.

Fawzy, F. I., & Fawzy, N. W. (1998). Group therapy in the cancer setting. *Journal of Psychosomatic Research*, *45*(3), 191–200.

Hargaden, H., & Sills, C. (2002). *Transactional analysis: A relational perspective*. New York: Brunner-Routledge.

Schore, A. N. (2009). Attachment trauma and the developing right brain: Origins of pathological dissociation. In *Dissociation and the dissociative disorders: DSM-V and beyond* (pp. 107–141). London: Routledge, Taylor & Francis Group.

Tangolo, A. E., & Massi, A. (2015). Essere Noi. *Percorsi di Analisi Transazionale*, *II*(1), 65–81.

Tuckman, B. W. (1965). Developmental sequence in small groups. *Psychological Bulletin*, *63*, 384–399.

Tuckman, B. W., & Jensen, M. A. C. (1977). Stages of small-group development revisited. *Group & Organization Studies*, *2*(4), 419–427.

Yalom, I. D. (2001). *The gift of therapy: An open letter to a new generation of therapists and their patients*. New York: HarperCollins.

Yalom, I. D., & Leszcz, M. (2005). *The theory and practice of group psychotherapy* (5th ed.). New York: Basic Books (Originally published in 1970).

4

INTERSUBJECTIVITY AND THE GROUP AS EMOTIONAL REGULATOR

Our nervous systems – as Stern points out – are constructed to be captured by the nervous systems of others, so that we can experience others *as if* from within their skin, as well as from within our own. A sort of direct feeling route into the other person is potentially open and we resonate with and participate in their experiences, and they in ours (Stern, 2004, p. 76).

The bonds we experience during our first years of life structure our brain and influence our choice of partner, our parenting style, our ability to deal with life's obstacles, and our levels of resilience and hope. Today we know the unconscious is not a static deposit of buried and silent memories. In fact, its nature is deeply relational: an unconscious mind communicates with another unconscious mind through non-verbal language, right brain to right brain (Schore, 1994). Brains synchronize in real time and interact spontaneously with each other through quick emotional messages. Schore uses the term *synchrony* (from the Greek: *Syn* – together – and *chronos* – time) to underline that this two-way communication happens at the same time. This concept is related to the idea of a physiological bond, a reciprocal affective exchange, aimed at the transmission and co-regulation of emotions. Simultaneously measuring the cerebral activity of two people during an instance of interpersonal communication demonstrated that an individual alters their emotional reactions depending on their partner's alterations of theirs, thus generating synchrony between their own right parietal cortex and their partner's (Dumas, Nadel, Soussignan, Martinerie, & Garnero, 2010). These studies highlight how brain synchronization in the right temporo-parietal junction is activated during social interactions and it is involved in attention development, perceptive awareness, recognition of facial and vocal cues, as well as other empathic skills.

Emotional right brain to right brain communication is also at the basis of attachment dynamics between child and caregiver, and it structures the ability of the child to regulate affection. In terms of development, the most important benefits are related to the fact that caregivers, thanks to their syntonization and synchronization skills, are able to identify the children's needs and thus act in a way that improves the child's chances of survival. Our species' young lacks an extensive brain development; it is only their ability to syntonize with the caregiver's mind

DOI: 10.4324/9781003215547-5

states that allows the child to establish fresh neuronal connections which will lead them to broaden their positive emotional states, control the negative ones, and develop self-regulation skills.

The moments the caregiver syntonizes emotionally with the child are instances of communication between right brains. The right hemisphere "knows" reality through emotion, perceiving it unconsciously in its less obvious aspects, while the left hemisphere contributes in a conscious way to the causal and verbal understanding of events: thus, in the caregiver–child relationship, the implicit, non-verbal, emotional, and musical aspects are responsible for the development of the child's emotional regulation system.

Schore's work applies to psychotherapy of this neurobiological-interpersonal model of non-verbal attachment and emotional communication. In it, Schore illustrates how the quick, dynamic, and fluctuating sharing of emotional states between client and therapist accounts for an organized dialogue spanning only a few milliseconds. In this interactive matrix, both partners spontaneously match their states and at the same time regulate their social attention, excitement stimulation, and acceleration, in response to their partner's signals (Schore, 2003).

Several neuroscientific studies postulate that inter-brain communication between right brains aids the development of the adaptive skill of perceiving others' emotional states (Schore, 1994). They also claim that the right hemisphere interprets the mental state not only of its own brain, but also of others (Keenan, Rubio, Racioppi, Johnson, & Barnacz, 2005, p. 702). This inter-brain perspective operates not only within the context of one-on-one psychotherapy but also within group psychotherapy. Right brain to right brain synchronization happens within a group during spontaneous and shared emotional social interactions, especially during mutual regressions.

According to Shuren and Grafman (2002), the right hemisphere contains the representations of the emotional states associated with the individual's past experiences. When a person finds themselves in contexts that remind them of family situations, as it happens in group psychotherapy, the representations of past emotional experiences are retrieved from the right hemisphere and subsequently incorporated in the rational process. In the case of group psychotherapy, members share implicit experiences – sense of abandonment, shame, terror, and pain – and then cooperate between them to give meaning to those experiences. Thus, there is a repetitive movement taking place that goes from regression to progression, from right to left brain: Mutual regression (right brain) is followed by a synchronized displacement toward the left brain, in order to come to a more objective, abstract, and cognitive understanding of the intersubjective emotional dynamics that have occurred. This way, past emotional experiences gain access to the mentalization process, that is, the ability to comprehend one's own mental states as well as others' (Fonagy, Gergely, Jurist, & Target, 2002).

Emotional regulation within groups according to TA

Hargaden & Sills claim that therapists and group members communicate "right brain – right brain" while the group functions as a container, facilitating members' emotional regulation. The authors, in the chapter of *Transactional Analysis: A Relational Perspective* dedicated to group therapy (Hargaden & Sills, 2002), describe the change in Theresa, an anxious and talkative client who, thanks to the non-verbal exchanges with the group therapist, gradually learns to manage her anxieties and her fears, improving her relationships with other members. Through non-interpretative, emotional work, Theresa, during group regression, introjected both members and therapist as "'good enough' P_0 – [which determined] a step to the growth of her undeveloped self" (p. 144), while her C_0, properly mirrored and legitimized in her archaic needs, started to express her most authentic feelings. We can see, in this brief clinical example, how unconscious communication and emotional regulation are at the center of the change processes implicit in group psychotherapy. Regression within the group reaches each member's script protocols, "the bedrock within which we first learn what it is to be alive and involved with others" (Cornell, 2010, p. 119). These regressions provide a group context in which the leader explores with members the deepest of experiences, slipping in a time without thought or word, through countertransferential resonance. Regressions influence both the therapist's emotions and body, so a shared mirroring, a non-verbal emotional communication, is generated between members, as if both leader and members were "giving up" to the right brain, diving into those interpersonal dissociative mechanisms and influencing their codification. Sharing fragments of ego states gives back to each individual their right to belong to a community, conveying a sense of group OKness: The invisible glue that integrates the inner parts of the self and restores vitality to its relationships with others.

In transactional analysis, the intra-psychic and interpersonal dissociative processes can be confronted working with an integrated approach that merges relational and structural perspectives.

According to Little (2017), dissociation emerges during the first few years of life, when the child splits and represses aspects of the self in order to protect themselves from the traumatic experiences they are not yet able to process and to satisfy their hunger for recognition (Berne, 1961). In this case, to be introjected into implicit memory are not the single ego states but fragments of the interactions between self and caregiver, in the form of relational schemas, at the pre-symbolic level. An internal bond is generated between Parent and Child, a strong bond of loyalty to what Little defines as ego states relational units. The relational unity protects from fear of abandonment, from the dread of ending up in a black hole: at the end of the day, aren't negative strokes more acceptable than a lack of strokes? A painful relationship fraught with abandonment is better than no relationship at all. The script-bound, structured internalizations of relationships that are linked together as Child-Parent ego states relational units run the risk of being entombed and imprisoned in these structures, and thus they need to emerge so as to allow the dissociated self to come to life (Little, 2017, p. 13). In the therapy group, the intra-psychic impasse becomes a relational impasse, in which interactions with others are feared but also necessary to the Child ego state. These are the moments of group regression in which right brains are syntonized and synchronized, and the feared relationship experienced at the sub-symbolic level is repeated through projective transference (Hargaden & Sills, 2002). It is mostly clients suffering from borderline disorder who project primitive object relations onto others in an effort to maintain a coherent sense of self. This script protocol activation, based on the non-verbal, corporeal unconscious, allows access to the different mechanisms of intersubjective change. It allows members to go through a painful experience in order, after having processed it, to create new ways to relate to others. During regressive moments, primary relational schemas emerge and, in particular, dysregulated emotions such as shame – that are situated in the right brain – are activated. The primitive affects projected outside convey implicit transferences of transactions that are emotionally and physically exhausting and undermine the group's cohesion. During these collisions of minds, the ego states relational units manifest essentially through enactments, as we shall see in Chapter 13, and they are subsequently understood, with the help of the therapist, thanks to the emergence of introjective and transformative transferences (Hargaden & Sills, 2002). Clients are enriched by the introjection of the therapist's or more mature members' good objects and they learn to find and build new images of themselves through the encounter with significant "others." Thus, the group encourages the experience and exploration of affection, including dissociated or repressed emotions – hitherto defensively avoided – in order to allow members to transform them into adaptive emotions (Schore, 2020). Stuthridge (2012) described this work as "integrating the fractured self" (p. 239): a process of emotional transformation to which both client and therapist unconsciously participate in a series of exchanges between right and left brain. This way, group psychotherapy offers the opportunity to transform relational units, thus freeing the resources therein contained. During this process, the repeated relation will evolve into necessary relation, engendering a transformation of the ego states' different structures which will give way to emotional regulation.

On this matter, we would like to present a brief clinical example.

Alfonso, 35 years old, lawyer, second child, has an older brother he has always perceived as better loved and valued by his parents. Within the group, he often accuses other members of not making him feel welcomed and listened to enough. He tends to reframe the therapist's or other members' contributions interpreting their considerations as hostile and rejecting toward him.

For example, during the 20th session, a group member, Carla, talks about her struggle with having a constructive dialogue with her younger son, and Alfonso interacts with her, underlining how this boy might have a deep inferiority complex with respect to his brother. Toward the end of the session, Carla thanks Alfonso for helping her understand her son's hurt, which until that moment had remained in the shadows. To these words, Alfonso reacts immediately with anger and hostility, accusing Carla of being a bad mother and, most of all, of always having underestimated his intelligence:

> You realize I'm smart just now! What about before? I know you, like everyone else here after all, always thought of me as an idiot, never really believed in me, I'm a good lawyer! – and to the whole group – You should see me in court, you'd like my speeches.

Group members, as usual, are disoriented when faced with this gratuitous hostility. Some laugh awkwardly, others try to explain to Alfonso that he misunderstood Clara's words, as if often happens to many of them. While the therapist listens to Alfonso screaming, she feels a sense of shame and fear overcoming her body: she would only like for Alfonso to leave, she fantasizes of standing up and shutting that mouth, from which so much nonsense keeps tumbling out. She turns to look at Carla, who fell silent and turned pale, her fingers tightening their hold of the armrests, and her eyes fixated on the wall in front of her. Shame, anger, mockery, and humiliation are the emotions that accompany the group's regression and are felt by all members on a physical level. During those few, long but relentless minutes of silence, the therapist understands that her shame and terror – emotions which may be synchronized and syntonized with Clara's – represent Alfonso's projective transference. The unbearable experiences contained in his ego states relational units "must" be perceived by someone else in order for him to be freed from his torment. In his screams, we can catch a glimpse of the struggle of an entire life spent trying to protect himself from humiliation and lack of recognition from his family, a Child's fear hiding behind an angry and violent Parent, the exhausting inner dialogue between a Victim and his Persecutor (Karpman, 1968) bonded in a loyalty pact difficult to break. Only when the therapist asks Alfonso how he is feeling, the group feels a greater sense of relief. This beneficial effect does not come from the therapist's words, but from her understanding of what was happening inside of her and her recovered ability to face Alfonso, conquering her fear. Carla's emotional intensity eases, and she can finally express her terror and helplessness, emotions she used to feel during her childhood when she often heard her violent father screaming. Thus, the repeated relation gives way to the necessary relation, so that each individual "can attend to the vulnerable self with its unfulfilled need for growth and development" (Little, 2011, p. 30).

Working on the pre-verbal needs of members' Child ego states also means working on their defenses and resistances to satisfy those needs. Alfonso describes his guilt for being responsible for Carla's pain and fear, and other members describe the intense emotional reactions they had to Alfonso's anger and hostility. Regressing to their original script protocol grants members the powerful possibility to directly get in touch with the ego states relational units, that is, those dissociated aspects pushing to emerge to consciousness and be integrated in the right brain's self. This process can be seen as an adaptive regression that favors the emergence of new integrations between ego states, a new level of group intimacy and new transformative transferences.

During the first year in group, Alfonso fails in his efforts to be accepted, welcomed, and respected, persisting in adopting irritating and frustrating behaviors. In time, the continuous feedback from members will help him really look at himself and better understand the impact his behaviors have on the people around him. He will then become able to connect what happens within the group with the interpersonal difficulties he experiences outside. "I'm paranoid" he will state after a year in group therapy, when he will be finally able to see himself from the outside, as an integrated and integrating Adult: in doing so, Alfonso will manifest a self-awareness he did not possess before and an understanding of the relational value of his behaviors and his Child's unexpressed needs. The implicit mechanisms that helped Alfonso learn about his interpersonal distortions can be found in self-observation and members' feedback, two elements Yalom sees as fundamental in his interpersonal approach we have already mentioned.

Alfonso and the group will come out of these experiences with a new strength, thanks to the shared awareness that expressing oneself, enacting the most terrifying objects without experiencing, or causing embarrassment, rejection, reproach, and judgment; this allows to psychically digest what before was unbearable. This is how the group becomes a mental container in which it is possible to introject the new ego states: these, along with the integration of fresh neural networks, will in turn integrate and change, becoming more and more coherent, flexible, articulated, and differentiated.

Intersubjectivity and reflecting on "we"

What makes group treatment particularly effective for deconfusion work – and thus for a deep psychodynamic therapy – is, as we have just seen, the implicit level of members' emotional learning. Clients with alexithymia, bipolar disorder, phobic personalities, and non-substance addictions all find a great relief in group therapy, apparently even without actively participating, that is, even just through purely listening sessions, in which clients learn from others' work. That is why it is important that groups be mixed, composed of clients with different psychic capacities and psychopathologies. The shared work of building new narrations engenders a new language that evolves with experience and provides a structure for cognitive processing, emotional regulation, and the ability to reflect on one's own experiences. This (subjective and objective) mirroring grants permission to members to express their feelings; it gives them the impression of being recognized amidst the intimacy of their own pain and suffering, as never before in their lives; it gives them the impression that abhorred thoughts, kept hidden for so long and perceived as a threat, are normal and familiar to others as well. Clients with alexithymia, bipolar disorder, phobic personalities, and personality disorders, while in group, experience strong emotions such as fear, anger, and a sense of exclusion. Old traumas are reenacted, with the same old strategies, and the therapist's calm reaction offers the mirroring that is necessary to collectively give meaning to the symptom, and the illness. In group, emotions are not recounted as in individual therapy, but they are directly experienced in the here-and-now because the presence of other members is a threat in and of itself. The terrifying internal objects are projected onto the group and the therapist, and the latter has enough time to reflect and try to undertake an emotional regulation work similar to that of the caregiver to the newborn, as we have seen earlier. The client's Child is placated because their emotions were "chewed" by the therapist and sometimes by better integrated group members. The therapeutic efficacy of group therapy does not originate from verbal interactions or cognitive intuition, but from emotional and relational mechanisms contained within the script protocol, as well as from the interactive regulation implicit in all members' right brains. Within the group, clients learn that, as we have observed in the aforementioned dialogue, no man is an island and to live means to recognize ourselves as part of a wide network of relations, both real and symbolic, which substantiate us and connect us to the world. The client's ego is then resized in its pretensions, having satisfied its innate need to be a part of something bigger than itself.

Mirror neurons help us understand this shared interpersonal space based on the correspondence between the meaning of one's own actions and feelings and the meaning of others' experiences: emotions and actions conveyed by others are perceived in one's own body through a mechanism that Vittorio Gallese (2005) defined as embodied simulation. The mirror neurons theory paves the way for the understanding of intersubjectivity as a pre-verbal condition starting from common neuronal mechanisms. When lacking in stimuli from an intersubjective matrix, the human identity dissolves or deforms. It is through the many interactions with others – which represent the weave and substance of one's own life – that personality dynamics are changed and perpetuated. According to Ammaniti and Gallese (2014), intersubjectivity is a fundamental human need which responds to the necessity, on one hand, of being able to read others' feelings and intentions, and, on the other, of keeping in touch with oneself, keeping one's own sense of cohesion and identity thanks to our peers' gaze.

According to Daniel Stern (2004), the concept of intersubjectivity helps us understand the characterizing dynamics of psychotherapeutic groups: it encourages group formation, enriches its functioning, and assures its cohesion. The need to orientate oneself intersubjectively within the group space causes the client to mobilitate their own individual behavior in order to foster intimate relationships or enact archaic script patterns, in case the intersubjective movements are met with obstacles. Indeed, intersubjectivity can be modulated and promoted but also opposed. Disturbances to intersubjectivity within a group emerge easily: the capacity of the therapy group to become a space of reflection, the "work group," is threatened by the "basic-assumption group" (Bion, 1959), as we have seen in Chapter 2. The dialectics between work groups and basic-assumption groups, between integrating and confusive dynamics, the synchronized displacement from rational left brain to emotional, unconscious right brain might allow the emergence of hidden forces, at the intra-psychic level, that would aid clients in understanding themselves in a relational context. Basic assumptions can be observed in facial expressions, gestures, posture, and people's looks while they interact with each other, and they all constitute the protomental system, in which mental and physical levels are still undifferentiated. From a TA point of view, the protomental system represents the script protocol. Basic assumptions stem from this system, which, as we have mentioned earlier, is closely related to corporeal processes: Other's intense past experiences are not verbalized but directly perceived within the body (embodied simulation) as if they were one's own. Emotions and actions observed within the group are simulated by clients in order to be understood through an immediate and unconscious process; intersubjectivity becomes intercorporeity. This way, empathy can be intended as an immediate perception of the Other's corporeity and deep emotions. It allows members to create an intersubjective affective bond and, at the same time, to maintain a clear distinction between the self and the Other.

Berne, too, well ahead of his time, mentioned a biological need pushing human beings to enter into a group, to experiment with social contact, even in its primitive forms: the need to keep active certain areas of the brain through external stimulation (Berne, 1963). Sitting in a circle, members look at each other and mirror each other, trying to maintain the sense of cohesion of one's own identity that sometimes gets lost due to the intense primordial anguish in which the group is steeped, causing feelings of depersonalization, especially in clients suffering from personality disorders. However, if the therapist is able to strike, within the group, a balance between the capacity to keep in touch with unconscious emotional and sensorial experiences and the capacity to put these experiences into words, in time, we can expect the symptom to change into an intelligible language, a language that can be shared and processed by all members through empathy (Rugi, 2004).

Foulkes used a suggestive image when referring to the group leader: "I feel like a conductor, but I don't know in the least what the music is which will be played" (Foulkes, 1975, p. 292). The concept of *Physis*, understood by Berne as a natural force which leads human beings to grow, make progress, and improve despite adversities, is of great help to the group therapist. They will trust the fact that in the group lay the basis of intersubjectivity and social living, which give way to new visions and scenarios. They will let members experience in the moment their own story, a story that is worth being told, shared, respected, and valued; they will head the work group activities and will be, at the same time, the expression of the opposing forces, always careful to let the connection between affective and rational life emerge and be processed by the group.

To be a group therapist means "to have the capacity to inhabit a condition of uncertainty, in order to avoid saturating and blocking the process with a rather premature attribution of meaning"[1] (Neri, n.d., p. 9); the skills to lead the group through the field of primitive emotions, games, and life forces, in order for its members to learn to interact with others not from any of the points of the dramatic triangle, but within a shared reciprocity. The group therapist can teach clients to be more and more authentic and humane because they themselves keep learning from the stories of interweavings and encounters that make each group unique and teach them to look at each member as an opportunity for growth and healing for everyone involved. Certainly, this openness to learning and dealing with uncertainty implies "giving up the hope of Santa Claus," to use Berne's metaphor (1966, p. 229), and other childhood idealizations. Thus, the end of therapy will be marked by forgiveness, acceptance of life for what it is and a healthy sense of humor.

As Tangolo puts it

> If one has an integrated and integrating Adult, the mourning process for the loss of Santa Claus will have been completed and the patient will be able to use humor – which Berne identifies as one of the healthy characteristics – with his therapist.
>
> (Tangolo, 2015, p. 145)

Note

1 My translation.

References

Ammaniti, M., & Gallese, V. (2014). *La nascita dell'intersoggettività: Lo sviluppo del sé tra psicodinamica e neurobiologia*. Milano: Raffaello Cortina.

Berne, E. (1961). *Transactional analysis in psychotherapy: A systematic individual and social psychiatry*. New York: Grove Press.

Berne, E. (1963). *The structure and dynamics of organizations and groups.* New York: Grove Press.

Berne, E. (1966). *Principles of group treatment.* New York: Grove Press.

Bion, W. (1959). *Experiences in groups.* New York: Basics Books.

Cornell, W. F. (2010). Whose body is it? Somatic relations in script and script protocol. In R. G. Erskine (Ed.), *Life scripts: A transactional analysis of unconscious relational patterns* (pp. 101–125). London: Karnac.

Dumas, G., Nadel, J., Soussignan, R., Martinerie, J., & Garnero, L. (2010). Inter-brain synchronization during social interaction. *PLoS One, 5*(8), e12166. doi:10.1371/journal.pone.0012166

Fonagy, P., Gergely, G., Jurist, E., & Target, M. (2002). *Affect regulation, mentalization, and the development of the self.* New York: Other Press.

Foulkes, S. H. (1975/1990). The leader in the group. In *Selected papers of S. H. Foulkes: Psychoanalysis and group analysis.* London: Karnac.

Gallese, V. (2005). Embodied simulation: From neurons to phenomenal experience. *Phenomenology and Cognitive Science, 4*, 23–48.

Hargaden, H., & Sills, C. (2002). *Transactional analysis: A relational perspective.* London: Brunner-Routledge.

Karpman, S. (1968). Fairy tales and script drama analysis. *Transactional Analysis Bulletin, 7*(26), 39–43.

Keenan, J. P., Rubio, J., Racioppi, C., Johnson, A., & Barnacz, A. (2005). The right hemisphere and the dark side of consciousness. *Cortex, 41*(5), 695–704. doi:10.1016/S0010-9452(08)70286-7

Little, R. (2011). Impasse clarification within the transference-countertransference matrix. *Transactional Analysis Journal, 41*(1), 23–38. doi:10.1177/036215371104100106

Little, R. (2017). Ego state relational units and resistance to change. *Transactional Analysis Journal, 36*, 7–19. doi:10.1177/036215370603600103

Neri, C. (n.d.). *Presentazione del metodo e della tecnica del social dreaming.* Relazione sui Workshops tenuti a Lem-al-dar, Mauriburg, Raissa e Clarice Town. Retrieved from www.claudioneri.it/wp-content/uploads/2013/05/presentazione-del-metodo-e-della-tecnica-del-social-dreaming.pdf

Rugi, G. (2004). *Empatia e intersoggettività nella psicoterapia di gruppo: Condivisione del dolore e neuroni specchio.* Retrieved from www.funzionegamma.it/empatia-e-inter soggettivita-nella-psicoterapia-di-gruppo-condivisione-del-dolore-e-neuroni-specchio/

Schore, A. N. (1994). *Affect regulation and the origin of the self: The neurobiology of emotional development.* Hillsdale, NJ: Erlbaum.

Schore, A. N. (2003). *Affect regulation and the repair of the self.* New York: W.W. Norton.

Schore, A. N. (2020). Forging connections in group psychotherapy through right brain-to-right brain emotional communications. Part 1: Theoretical models of right brain therapeutic action. Part 2: Clinical case analyses of group right brain regressive enactments. *International Journal of Group Psychotherapy, 70*(1), 29–88. doi:10.1080/00207284.2019.1682460

Shuren, J. E., & Grafman, J. (2002). The neurology of reasoning. *Archives of Neurology, 59*(6), 916. doi:10.1001/archneur.59.6.916

Stern, D. (2004). *The present moment in psychotherapy and everyday life.* New York: W.W. Norton.

Stuthridge, J. (2012). Traversing the fault lines: Trauma and enactment. *Transactional Analysis Journal, 42*, 238–251. doi:10.1177/036215371204200402

Tangolo, A. E. (2015). *Psychodynamic psychotherapy with transactional analysis: Theory and narration of a living experience* (A. Iozzelli & K. Jones, Trans.). London: Karnac (Originally published in 2010).

5

CLIENT SELECTION AND GROUP COMPOSITION

In order for therapy groups to work well, it is important to establish the principles of group composition through a clear set of criteria, which in turn allow for a careful selection of the clients better suited for this type of treatment.

The research on therapy groups does not offer any specific guidelines on how to select clients, so, in order to choose aptly, we have to trust our intuition and the years of personal experience. The composition of a heterogeneous, open group requires a clinical reading of a client's needs and motivations to change, as well as their ability to deal with the "enactment" of impulses in the context of treatment. Once we have selected the clients, we will move on to decide which group might be more helpful to which client.

Inclusion criteria

According to Berne "In practice, however, almost any patient can be introduced to a treatment group after proper preparation" (Berne, 1966, p. 4). Berne preferred heterogeneous groups, which better reflected the regular social context. Foulkes (1975), too, believed that clients apt for individual therapy may also be for group therapy, and, in some cases, he even purported that group therapy might be useful for those clients for whom individual therapy had been considered unsuitable.

Today, studies confirm that not only group therapy works, but it is also as efficient as individual therapy (Burlingame, Fuhriman, & Mosier, 2003): indeed, it has proven to be even more efficient than one-on-one therapy in providing social learning and support, as well as developing a web of social interactions (Graham, Annis, Brett, Venesoen, & Clifton, 1996). The pathologies of this day and age are in many cases connected to the difficulties in building intimate and satisfying relationships (see Introduction). Group therapy is the therapy of choice for these types of pathologies, and thus, in agreement with Berne and Foulkes, in assessing the inclusion criteria of group psychotherapy, we may take into consideration all clients who are able to establish and sustain a therapeutic relationship. Another inclusion criterion is provided by the client's motivation. Some studies have indeed shown that the more motivated the client – that is, the more they expect group therapy to be useful – the more therapy will prove to be useful (Frank &

    DOI: 10.4324/9781003215547-6

Frank, 1991). Additionally, the client's willingness to take the risk of giving and receiving feedback, and to open up to self-disclosure, with the ensuing emotional involvement, also increases the efficacy of treatment (Melnick & Rose, 1979). A thorough preparation of the client to face group therapy might also contribute to strengthen their motivation and their intention of putting themselves out there assuming all the risks that might entail.

Del Corno and Lang list the following inclusion criteria for heterogeneous, open, long-term groups:

1 The most acute problems manifest in the area of regular interpersonal relationships.
2 Clients are capable of opening up and communicate with people who are different than them.
3 The excessive intellectualization would thwart any attempt at individual therapy.
4 Clients feel overcome by such intense feelings which, being unable to contain or put into thought, they short circuit into somatic symptoms.
5 Clients run the risk of getting stuck into a regressive transference or they may not be able to bear the intimacy of a dual relationship, or they may engender countertransference reactions difficult to deal with in a dual therapy setting (Del Corno & Lang, 2004, pp. 32–33).[1]

Exclusion criteria

On the other hand, when a client who lacks motivation expresses a clear-cut refusal to join a therapy group, the therapist should desist from persuading them, since this would mean to ally themselves with their Adapted Child.

Maria, a client who had been undergoing individual therapy for about three years, during which she had managed to report a violent husband and separate from him, had answered with a blunt "no" to the therapist's invite to enter a therapy group – said invite being motivated by her enormous difficulties in establishing social relationships and by a deep-seated feeling of loneliness. This refusal, expressed with assertiveness, surprised the therapist in a positive manner: in fact, Maria used to express a dependent personality, with a strong Adapted Child who tended to indulge in others' requests, and felt usually quite reluctant to freely express her own ideas. For this reason, the therapist chose to welcome Maria's refusal, which meant to meet the needs of her Free Child, who had emerged unexpectedly after years of fear and repression. Maria appeared to regret what she regarded as a reckless answer and started stammering something like "but

---

if you feel like this would do me good, . . . I'm scared but." The therapist's encouragement to adhere to her needs and respect the fears of her Child, who had been always oppressed by "the adults" (her mother abandoned her when she was three years old and her father had always been rough and punitive toward her), strengthened Maria's capacity to freely express what she felt and, most of all, transformed her alliance with the therapist, which went from *necessary* and *functional* to the fight against the outside enemy, her husband, to *aware* and the product of a *free* choice. They moved forward, then, with individual therapy, which became more and more intimate and spontaneous. Maria proved herself more relaxed and in touch with her feelings, so much so that, about a year after that episode, it was Maria herself who directly asked the therapist to enter group therapy. At that point, she felt ready to face the group and answer affirmatively to the therapist's invite of a year before, not because she was adapting, but because she had chosen to trust the therapist.

Beside clients unmotivated to start group therapy, we have to exclude, as we would for individual therapy, those subjects suffering from severe psychosis, cerebropathy, sociopathy, or even subjects belonging to a rigid politic or religious ideology and prone to proselytism: these types of people need interventions aimed at containment more than processing. Nosographic classification is absolutely insufficient to determine inclusion or exclusion criteria for group therapy. Indeed, to a therapist that is careful about the ethical aspects of their work, the question should instead be which group might be more useful to a specific type of client. For clients who manifest antisocial behaviors, for example, the heterogeneous psychodynamic group is considered unsuitable. However, research has shown that there have been positive results with these types of clients in homogeneous intensive groups (Morgan & Winterowd, 2002). Homogeneous groups prove themselves immensely useful for other disorders such as drug or alcohol addiction (Strepparola, 2003). Clients suffering from severe forms of paranoia, before being inserted into a therapy group, should undergo a long one-on-one therapeutic treatment aimed at decontaminating their Adult ego state, in order to learn how to trust others: otherwise, they could easily run the risk of getting stuck into playing games such as "Now I Got You" or "Blemish," attacking the therapist or other group members, and denying any kind of Adult–Adult interaction. There are empirical studies on defections during the initial stages of group therapy, which suggest some important exclusion criteria (Yalom, 1966). In order to facilitate a healthy group process, it is of paramount importance to avoid bringing into the group clients who are very likely to suspend treatment. First of all, this will obviously safeguard clients at risk of dropping out. Second, it will also protect those who stay and might have negative reactions to the emptiness left behind so prematurely, before the development of a solid group cohesion.

Yalom found various causes that might push clients to end group treatment prematurely. Among the most important, he lists external factors, group deviancy, and problems of intimacy.

External factors

Every time a client expresses their intention of dropping out because of external factors, it is necessary to thoroughly assess the real existence of such factors (job changes, sudden losses, severe physical ailments, etc.), since in some cases, the drop out might be motivated by a defensive displacement caused by the client's Child, who might be perceiving the group as a threat and thus be terrified of it.

> After completing a three-year-long individual treatment, Valeria had joined a women-only group, which she had been attending for two months. The decision to face group therapy had been taken together with the therapist because of her inclination to establish competitive relationships with other women, both friends and colleagues. This problem had led her to change many jobs, and at the time of entering the group, she had been newly hired by a transport company, but her employer had already threatened to fire her because of her ceaseless fights with her female coworkers. During the first two months of group therapy, she had kept silent, listening to other members without sharing anything, frowning, at times snorting irritably, and, if confronted with her displays of annoyance, attributing them to her usual migraines.
>
> Nobody believed her when she announced her decision to leave the group because of a change in her husband's work schedule, which had been changed from a morning to an afternoon shift.
>
>> We don't know who we should leave our three-year-old daughter with when I have to come here once a week, since I'd have to be out of the house for four hours, and we don't have any grand-parents to leave her with, and a baby sitter would be too expensive. . . . Maybe I could go back to the individual therapy sessions in the morning.
>
> It was clear to both therapist and members that Valeria was shifting the negative emotions she felt about the group toward her husband's changed work schedule. The therapist tried to empathize with Valeria's fearful, angry Child (her mother was an unloving woman, who cared a lot about

her appearance and often frequented clubs and pubs, so much so that Valeria, in her adolescence, would avoid going out in fear of running into her in one of the places she used to go to with her friends), but she also manifested her firm refusal to go back to one-on-one sessions, since that would have enabled Valeria's belief of being incapable of facing the competitive nature of her relationships with other women. Moreover, if she had dropped out, the likeness of her being fired would have grown stronger, and that would have cost her a lot more, in terms of money and mental health, compared with a babysitter hired for merely four hours a week.

In this case, it was easy to uncover the true nature of the so-called external factors mentioned by Valeria, and this allowed the client to stay in the group, find the courage to face her own hostility and avoid getting fired. Other times it is not as easy to inquire with clients whether their request to drop out is connected to a real factor or is instead a resistance to venture into unfamiliar and hostile territory, conjuring up ancient fears and terrors. However, this is always an important task to be carried out with the utmost respect and attention toward the resistances of the subject in treatment.

Deviancy

Deviancy refers to those subjects who lack interpersonal sensitivity, who are unwilling to accept group rules and who show great difficulties in controlling their impulses. The mistake therapist often make with these subjects is to insert them into a group hoping to achieve better results, after experiencing a discouraging lack of progress in the individual setting. There are indeed many studies advocating the efficacy of group therapy in such cases (Leszcz, 1989). However, these studies argue that certain precautions need to be taken when inserting this type of subjects into the group, in order to avoid undermining the survival of the group itself. First, it is fundamental to placate their impulsive aspects and strengthen their observing Adult, delaying their entrance into the group so as to first allow them to benefit from pharmacological treatment and individual therapy. Additionally, it is necessary to accompany group therapy with individual sessions appropriately spaced in time, in order to create space for reflection and added containment. Finally, it is better not to insert more than two deviant subjects within a group that has been working for some time and in which several treatments have had a positive outcome. We will examine these subjects' characteristics more in depth within the chapter dedicated to personality disorders.

Intimacy problems

Such problems might emerge in opposite ways: on one hand, a withdrawal into oneself and a refusal to open up, or, on the other, an urgent need to disclose deeply intimate and delicate part of oneself, often related to childhood traumas, before the group has developed a strong cohesion. The Don't Be Close injunction belongs to many subjects who manifest difficulties in interpersonal relationships, and for these subjects, group therapy is especially recommended, but when this injunction is accompanied by a spontaneous emotionality strongly repressed by racked feelings, it prevails over all other injunctions: thus, lacking any kind of permission, the group might constitute a real threat.

A total lack of intimacy may predispose the subject to a compulsion to psychological games: they become inclined to see themselves as Victims, keeping silent and cultivating the hidden need for someone to invite them to speak, or launching in sterile, boring monologues lacking any real emotion.

These clients feel a deep anguish when in a group, fearing the possibility of losing their sense of self and being swallowed into an undifferentiated mass. Berne defined intimacy as a "game-free exchange of affective expression without covert exploitation" (Berne, 1966, p. 366).

This allows us to understand how a client with a strong Don't Be Close injunction may benefit a lot from group therapy, since the latter would become the first opportunity offered to them to overcome a rigid and limiting interpersonal relational model, based exclusively on games. However, instead of leaving this type of client alone, the therapist must help them – delicately and empathically – to calibrate their expressive and thus their relational model, in order to minimize the risk of the client of leaving treatment abruptly or becoming the group's scapegoat.

According to Dubois (1990), there is a deep connection between the therapist's capacity to integrate within themselves the client psychopathological aspects and the group's capacity to contain and integrate those same aspects. If the therapist set themselves up as a model of integration of all the shameful – or despicable, according to the client – components, then the group will be able to accept and integrate them as elements that belong to all human beings and can be shared. Tangolo writes: "Group therapy . . . is an extremely enriching experience, because it allows us to inhabit that interpersonal space of cognitive, emotional, and physical intimacy with other human beings, an intimacy we are less and less used to" (Marconcini, 2018, p. 28).[2]

As we have seen, there are no definite rules to select clients so as to ensure that the group works at its best. When group therapy is done in the proper way, defections are nonetheless always to be expected, because, otherwise, if the therapy group was characterized by the constant presence of all members, it might mean that the exclusion criteria have been applied too rigidly and the therapist might have avoided taking the risk of welcoming those clients with a higher possibility of dropping out, but for which group therapy would be an efficient treatment (Swiller, 2009). Believing that all clients, even the most troubled, are capable of improving their condition is at the basis of the ethical assumption "I'm OK – you're OK," and each transactional analyst should offer all clients, even the most troubled, the opportunity to avail themselves of this treatment, according to Berne's teachings. There are precautions that, as we have mentioned, may be taken in order to protect the individual client and the whole group, acting under the assumption that no criterion can fully appreciate the complexity of the subject who, entering the group, brings their story and their expectations: we cannot indeed entirely foresee how the baggage of the individual will interact with the interpersonal microcosm it will meet. Selecting which group might be useful for a specific client and which client might be useful for a specific group is the next necessary task a therapist will have to face after selecting clients, as we will see in the next paragraph.

Group composition

Therapy groups, as we have established, are kind of social microcosms, that is, miniature universes in which to learn how to be with others in new and constructive ways: the more heterogeneous the group, the more learning opportunities for its members. Group heterogeneity grants representation to the different groups of people inhabiting the world outside, thus providing members with some kind of experimental laboratory. When we talk about group heterogeneity, we are talking about different elements, including age, which may vary between 22 and 70 years. Broad as this spectrum may look, we have found that interacting with different generations provides clients with a better understanding of the script aspects characterizing the various stages of life, allowing them to view the actions, behaviors, and messages of parents, children, and siblings from a different angle. This possibility gives them a way out of their narrow perspective – a perspective that is contaminated by the Parent's prejudices and the Child's fears – and allows them to open up in order to explore and build a wider range of narratives.

Among other important elements typifying heterogeneity, we find gender identity: it is recommendable to have a balanced gender distribution, and in the event of this being an impossibility, it would be advisable to avoid the presence of only one man or only one woman in a group, opting instead for at least two members of the same gender. Education level, socioeconomic status, and professional role are also elements to be taken into consideration when we are referring to the group's heterogeneity.

Yalom's rule (Yalom & Leszcz, 2005), employed in the long-term psychodynamic therapy group, may help us pinpoint an adequate group composition: *heterogeneity for conflict areas* and *homogeneity for ego strength*. *Heterogeneity for conflict areas* is what we have just described, and involves gender, age, interpersonal difficulties, and the different models clients use to deal with hostility: there will be those who deal with it openly and those who tend to become passive and adapt to the needs of others.

Homogeneity relates to the clients' ability to tolerate anguish, to give and receive feedback, and to commit to the therapeutic process. It is also connected to the clients' willingness to leave behind their prejudices and the contamination of the Adult by the Parent and the Child. However, we know quite well that not all clients possess this ability. Clients suffering from serious personality disorders have limitations when it comes to the interpersonal field and adaptability, and thus need a setting that will support them in overcoming said limitations, also because their role within the group will be different from that of clients with a decontaminated Adult. While the latter might be more willing to process dynamics connected to intimacy and authenticity, clients suffering from serious disorders will have to deal with their discomfort at being in a room with other people, tolerating an extended interpersonal situation and trying to reflect on those emotions they would much prefer to act on immediately. The therapist should not insert more than two people affected by personality disorders within a group composed of seven to eight people, discerning from the beginning the dissonance that might ensue between these two people and other members: on one hand, it is necessary for the therapist to help clients with serious mental illness to tolerate anxiety, and, on the other, they must support other members in tolerating the aforementioned clients' requests during specific moments of the therapeutic process.

Oscar is a 35-year-old single man, suffering from borderline personality disorder, who has been in treatment for about three years. Oscar's entrance into the group proved itself to be very difficult, even if it was prepared by three years of individual psychotherapy and a pharmacological treatment prescribed by a psychiatrist with whom the group therapist is regularly in touch. In the course of the individual therapy process, Oscar had managed to get in touch with his lack of emotional regulation and had accepted the idea of taking medications, identifying the origin of his difficulties. At the same time, together with his therapist, he had decided to join a group in order to overcome his fear of intimacy with women. Thus, the therapist chose to insert Oscar into a group formed by "veterans," clients who have been attending the group for at least three years, who are able to react in a constructive manner to the emotional needs of a more vulnerable subject.

In group, at the very beginning, Oscar used to alternate long silences, full of yawns and looks at the clock, to moments of verbal hostility toward both the therapist and other group members. In particular, he used to berate the therapist for choosing the wrong group for him. In his opinion, he should have been inserted into a more problematic context, with more troubled and aggressive people: he would "get bored listening for two hours straight, without even a cigarette break, to the dull complaints of a couple of 'losers.'" These triangulations were often replied by Elena, a 47-year-old woman, who had also joined the group, four years before, with symptoms similar to Oscar's: verbal hostility, impulsiveness, and tendency to project her dissatisfaction on other members. Elena had changed a lot during the years and some of her symptoms had disappeared, developing instead a greater level of self-reflection and a better way of relating to people in terms of OKness, even if at times she might relapse into hostile behaviors. Faced with Oscar's belligerence, Elena kept her composure and seemed energized in trying to persuade him of the fact that his behavior hid a profound vulnerability, one she used to know very well, since she had gone through a similar process in the past. It was important for Elena to help Oscar insert himself into a new reality which he saw as a threat: "For me, it is like seeing parts of a past version of myself, and on one hand, I feel anger, while on the other, tenderness." In turn, other members supported Elena by giving her strokes in order to appreciate her changes and the strength she used with Oscar, but, unbeknownst to them, they were also supporting the therapist, who was afraid of getting from them an expulsive reaction to Oscar's arrogant behavior. Inserting a vulnerable client in a group considered mature enough does not ward off the therapist's worries, since, as we have seen before, this entrance is always a risk and may often lead to an unforeseeable turn of events. Even if Oscar threatened several times to leave the group, he never did, and Elena and the group's Parent was an invaluable container for Oscar's fearful, angry Child. Thus, he was able to continue to work on overcoming racket anger and get in touch with his sadness and fear of being abandoned.

This case helps us understand how it is paramount to pay attention to the levels of progress of all group members, especially when we insert new subjects who display obvious relational difficulties, precisely because the group climate tends to change swiftly with the entrance of a new member, and group cohesion might be lost. Additionally, we observed how the therapeutic factor of altruism was instrumental in solidifying Elena's changes and preventing Oscar from dropping out. The most altruistic clients, those most willing to commit, put themselves out there, and take risks, will not only make progress in their treatment, but also be able to support the less altruistic and cooperative clients in their work of interpersonal and intrapersonal exploration.

Conclusions

The composition of a therapy group proves to be a complex task, at the intersection of several social and cultural factors, on different levels. Paying attention to these levels helps the therapist to fulfill this task, with the firm understanding that the perfect combination of members does not exist. Client selection before entrance into the group is important to avoid random assignment. Often, therapists form a group considering the availability of the clients they oversee in one-on-one therapy, and if their number is small, the choice might not take into account the criteria of selection and composition we have mentioned earlier.

It is crucial to "think" clients before they join the group, to "keep" them in mind, imagine their hypothetical reactions to their encounter with others and the others' reactions to this new client: to "think" clients and to imagine them in action within the group, while at the same time being open and flexible to the unpredictable, ready to welcome what will happen in the real encounter between who is listening and who is narrating themselves. Eshkol Nevo, in his splendid novel *Three Floors Up*, proclaims:

> The three floors of the psyche do not exist inside us at all! Absolutely not! They exist in the air between us and someone else, in the space between our mouths and the ears we are telling our story to. And if there is no one there to listen – there is no story.

(Nevo, 2017, p. 286)

Thus, to "think" the client before inserting them into a group means to keep together their contradictions and fragments, hoping that "that group," with its stories and its ability to listen, will help them find a sense of self in order to integrate the needs of the Child, the most adaptive and flexible parts of the Adult, and those of the Containing and Nurturing Parent.

Notes

1 My translation.
2 My translation.

References

Berne, E. (1966). *Principles of group treatment*. New York: Grove Press.
Burlingame, G. M., Fuhriman, A., & Mosier, J. (2003). The differential effectiveness of group psychotherapy: A meta-analytic perspective. *Group Dynamics: Theory, Research, and Practice*, 7(1), 3–12. doi:10.1037/1089-2699.7.1.3
Del Corno, F., & Lang, M. (2004). *Trattamenti in setting di gruppo*. Milano: Franco Angeli.
Dubois, C. (1990). Psychotérapie de groupe en pratique privée. *Revue de Psychotérapie Psychoanalytique de Groupe*, *14*.
Foulkes, S. H. (1975). *Group analytic psychotherapy: Methods and principles*. London: Gordon & Breach.
Frank, J., & Frank, J. (1991). *Persuasion and healing: A comparative study of psychotherapy*. Baltimore: Johns Hopkins University Press.
Graham, K., Annis, H., Brett, P., Venesoen, P., & Clifton, R. (1996). A control field trial of group versus individual cognitive behavioral training for relapse prevention. *Addiction*, *91*, 1127–1139. doi:10.1046/j.1360-0443.1996.91811275.x

Leszcz, M. (1989). Group psychotherapy of the characterologically difficult patient. *International Journal of Group Psychotherapy*, *39*, 311–335.

Marconcini, A. (2018). Intervista ad Anna Emanuela Tangolo. *Percorsi di Analisi Transazionale*, *V*(4), 23–31.

Melnick, J., & Rose, G. (1979). Expectancy and risk-taking propensity. *Small Group Behavior*, *10*, 389–401.

Morgan, R., & Winterowd, C. (2002). Interpersonal process-oriented group psychotherapy with offender populations. *International Journal of Offender Therapy and Comparative Criminology*, *46*, 466–482.

Nevo, E. (2017). *Three floors up* (S. Silverston, Trans.). New York: Other Press.

Strepparola, G. (2003). *Operare nelle dipendenze patologiche*. Milano: Franco Angeli.

Swiller, H. I. (2009). Psychodynamic group therapy. In G. O. Gabbard (Ed.), *Textbook of psychotherapeutic treatments* (pp. 625–40). Washington, DC: American Psychiatric Publishing.

Yalom, I. D. (1966). A study of group therapy dropouts. *Archives of General Psychiatry*, *14*(4), 393. doi:10.1001/archpsyc.1966.01730100057008

Yalom, I. D., & Leszcz, M. (2005). *The theory and practice of group psychotherapy* (5th ed.). New York: Basic Books (Originally published 1970).

6

SETTING

Set and setting

The set is the physical space where a group meets. It must entail a physical or virtual room where there is space for everyone. If the group meets online, it is necessary to use digital tools in order to allow clients and therapist to see each other. If the set is physical, the clients' seats must be arranged in a circle so that everyone might see the others' faces. Clients sit on chairs, armchairs, or sofas: we believe it would be inappropriate for them to sit on rugs because this might prove difficult for elder clients or clients with reduced mobility, while it remains fundamental for all of them to sit at the same height and at the right distance between each other, so as to feel in touch but not overwhelmed by the overhanging or intrusive presence of another. The place where the group meets must be sober and welcoming in order to allow people from different cultural and geographical backgrounds to feel at ease. The room is the therapist's environment and as such it can be decorated according to their aesthetic taste and personality, albeit without exaggerating.

With regard to this matter, Tangolo (2010) wrote:

> It's like saying: this office and my clothes define me; here I have my music, my colours, but you can have your own space on the scene. Indeed, if sounds, perfumes, music, or colours are too intense, it is as if they do not allow space for the other, so that he [they] cannot be with us as a protagonist, only as a spectator.
>
> A psychotherapist's office is not the stage for an actor who recites monologues before the spectator-client: on the contrary, it can be a stage where one can find a protagonist role and interact with a person who listens to us and creates a space for the other person to express himself [themselves].

(p. 48)

The room works as a container, a safe place, and group members usually prefer not to change the environment where the meetings take place. Even the spatial disposition of chairs, armchairs, and sofas is important in order to create a welcoming

DOI: 10.4324/9781003215547-7

environment, and it is the therapist's duty to guarantee the same amount of comfort to all members.

Besides the set, the setting is composed of all the rules and the administrative, ethical, and relational agreements that are necessary to safely lead a therapy group. Therefore, in psychotherapy, by setting, we mean every rule established by the therapist and every agreement with clients, which clearly defines the nature of the relationship between them.

Rule-inspiring principles

The group setting must be built on the assumption that the group works as a family, with its table, its power dynamics and the affection, it is necessary to feed younger members and shield them until they are able to define themselves as individuals outside their family. In TA, we would say that the group-container is akin to the Parent-container: like a protective uterus allowing clients a safe development before "being born" – opening up – to new relationships where the differentiation process makes it possible for everyone involved to have more authentic, less unilateral exchanges. The parental nucleus in a group setting is represented both by the therapist and by the group itself, with all the rules and habits that make up the safety structure necessary for defining the self.

The basic principle underlying this type of psychotherapy is that within the group, there is space for everyone and everyone has the same rights. Everyone is owed respect and recognition, and violence toward others is forbidden, including the verbal kind. Therefore, bringing in weapons is forbidden as well. Moreover, members cannot join a session when under the influence of drugs or alcohol. All religious and political beliefs, as well as opinions on life, are welcomed.

In our groups, the regulatory principles of the relationships between members are not rendered explicit from the beginning or fixed in a rigid set of rules, as in some kinds of constitutional chart. We deem it preferable for principles to be defined during the course of treatment and by the therapist themselves, who embodies a vision of life in harmony with both "human rights" and the ethical code of transactional analysis organizations. We also believe that letting clients express conflictual opinions or points of view on values, ethics, and principles might be an excellent opportunity to explore the specific qualities of their introjected Parent.

Because of the nature of values and their significance in human life, and in order to guarantee the respect and rights of each person, it is necessary to identify clear guidelines of behavior, which are strictly linked to values. Ethical principles are derived from values and are intended as an indication of how to practice, in order to promote the well-being, development, and growth of a person. They are prescriptive and offer criteria for ethical behavior. Using values as the starting point, it is possible to determine a set of ethical principles. The principal ones are: Respect, Empowerment, Protection, Responsibility, and Commitment in relationship (EATA Ethical Code, 2011, p. 6).

Relationship ethics

The therapist's ethical perspective, prone to giving value to every opinion and to recognize each individual as a carrier of values, should emerge from their behavior and constitute the premise of an environment that is respectful of differences. An attention to values should transpire first of all from the therapist's lifestyle, from a coherence between what is said and what it actually is. Obviously, it is necessary that they express their political or religious beliefs soberly, but at the same time, they should not hide when confronted with explicit questions from their clients.

That said, it is advisable to remember that the group is not a house of parliament where every decision must be put to a vote. Some decisions are under the therapist's sole responsibility, such as those related to the time and place of meetings, the fee, breaks distribution, the conditions to join the group, the eventuality of a client having to drop out, or a client reaching the end of treatment.

The structure composed by the person of the therapist and the setting involves an agreement on the time and place of the sessions, as well as on the general rules of sharing a space with others. Also, part of the agreement on the setting is the members' acceptance of a mutual learning system related to how they express emotions, deal with psychic pain, and share opinions on existential matters.

Organizational models

We use two setting models, which combine individual and group therapies. In model A, clients join a group only after a period of individual therapy, with a two-hour group session once a week, which replaces the one-on-one meeting with the therapist. Clients gain access to this stage of treatment after they worked, during the course of the previous individual sessions, on building up the therapeutic alliance and on decontamination. The latter aims to foster acknowledgment, in clients, of the source of their problems, as well as acquisition of the necessary skills to deal with their most relevant symptoms from an Adult ego state. During the course of group therapy, upon a client's request, the therapist may grant an individual session, the contents of which will be shared with the group jointly by therapist and client, since the whole group participates in the analysis process of the members' script: thus, this sharing takes on a co-therapeutic function.

In model B, the group setting combines with the individual one, and therapy takes place in four sessions a month, alternating individual and group sessions. Here, too, each client may access group therapy after a period of individual treatment, but, for the entirety of their time in group, they will have two individual sessions a month with the therapist to discuss more in depth what they are experiencing in group and to be supported in dealing with their emotional difficulties. Several studies suggest that this type of setting is particularly apt for clients suffering from personality disorders, such as borderline or narcissistic disorders (see Chapter 15) In our experience we do not have definitive proof that using different models yields significantly different results, even if it would be undoubtedly useful to conduct a comparative study on the effects on clients of the different models.

From our standpoint, the therapist's specific training and their greater familiarity and confidence in dealing with one model might justify a preference of one over the other. Generally, we could say that, in the case of model A, it is as if the therapist, by taking away individual support, was inviting the client to take a major leap forward in their personal growth, while in the case of model B, the same growth would take place in a more gradual manner by maintaining an individual space along with the group sessions.

Basic rules

There is only one condition we require clients to accept before joining a group and this concerns confidentiality. Those who are able to take this responsibility on themselves may join the group. Besides that, we invite clients to stay for a minimum of six months and to dedicate three sessions to the separation process in case they decide to end group therapy prematurely. Clients are also required to accept giving and receiving feedback during sessions. These are, obviously, general guidelines and not fixed rules. A fixed rule, in fact, constitutes a parental prescription which implies an adaptive response. General guidelines, instead, involve a number of propositions, communicated Adult to Adult, which clients are invited to embrace after they have understood their purpose within treatment. Violating a fixed rule is a transgression, while failing to uphold a contract formulated Adult to Adult is a decision which might be verbalized as a disagreement. Indeed, we find it useful that clients, after they have adapted to the setting, train their Adult thought: this is a formative dimension of group therapy which allows members to understand, in time, how some guidelines are respectful to others and beneficial for themselves.

Time, absences, and lateness

Group sessions usually last either 90 minutes or 2 hours. Some members are especially punctual, while others tend to be often late. In this case, too, we deem it useful not to give an explicit rule, and instead analyze members' behaviors and the impact these have on others. Some people become annoyed at seeing others come late, while others are delighted because they have the pleasure to have more time and space to talk. With regard to absences, we believe it convenient to analyze the motivations behind them and consider them as supervision and research material. For example, too high a number of absences is an issue worth exploring further, since it indicates scarce motivation to therapy and scarce cohesion in the group process.

A clinical example in the structuring of time in group

Terry is worried, and she lacks the time to talk about herself in group and fears the others' competition. After having thought about it for a while, she submits to the rest of the group the idea of dividing up their speaking time equally, so that each member might speak without taking time away from others and without having to fight to be heard. It might be easier to be "alone together," says Terry, who is afraid of any kind of competition. It was very useful to explore the world of rules Terry made up in order to avoid confrontation and contact, whenever the situation ran the risk of becoming competitive.

Unwritten norms

During the course of his extensive studies and rich clinical experience on groups, Yalom writes highly encouraging pages on the emergence within groups of unwritten norms, often determined by the therapist's modeling function and the long-time members' greater authority.

We find it useful to quote his conclusions on the matter:

> To summarize: every group evolves a set of unwritten rules or norms that determine the procedure of the group. The ideal therapy group has norms that permit the therapeutic factors to operate with maximum effectiveness. Norms are shaped both by the expectations of the group members and by the behavior of the therapist. The therapist is enormously influential in norm setting – in fact, it is a function that the leader cannot avoid. Norms constructed early in the group have considerable perseverance. The therapist is thus well advised to go about this important function in an informed, deliberate manner.
>
> (Yalom & Leszcz, 2005, pp. 167–168)

In one such groups, "elder" members had established an unwritten norm concerning the ritual cigarette they would smoke outside after a session. Those who did not stay, avoiding this ritual of inclusion among peers, were refused consideration during group interactions. This fact was brought to the therapist's attention when one of the outcasts noted during a session how members would use that specific moment to comment on the session that had just ended, thus violating the explicit agreement they had with the therapist not to talk about the group outside sessions. The group member who violated the unwritten norm was considered for a long time a "killjoy" who betrayed a pact with his peers.

Fees

When it comes to fees, we advise to set the group up as having a regular monthly fee and this fee has to be paid by each member regardless of their attendance record. Generally speaking, every choice the therapist makes with regard to fees implies the risk of games, but this risk seems to us to be never entirely avoidable. If we decided to let members pay only for the sessions they attended to, there would be a risk of facilitating absences and encouraging avoidant behavior. If we decided that members must also pay for unwarranted or unreported absences, we might find ourselves arguing on which absences are warranted for work or health reasons, and which ones are not, or on the validity of certain reasons members give for not reporting their absence. If the fee is made up of a fixed monthly quota paid in advance, on one hand, the therapist risks less when managing the economic contract, but, on the other, they lose the possibility of analyzing the hooks for games which, when it comes to economic matters, always convey important elements of a relationship: anger, envy, greed, a desire to trick the therapist, the pretense to be "saved," or taken care of like a child.

In one such occasion, a group member, Lia, decides to drop out declaring to the others she cannot afford therapy anymore. During the exchange, all members point out, instead, that it would be really important for her to go on with the treatment. Another member, Andrea, tries to persuade her to stay offering to pay her fees for three months. At that point, the group confronts Andrea on the reason behind this striking offer. We find out that, for Andrea, the loss of Lia would be a source of grief. When Andrea was a child, he had put it on himself to avoid his parents' separation, which, instead, had been fraught with conflict, leaving him alone and unhappy. When Andrea becomes able to connect the two events, he makes a great leap forward in his treatment.

Interactions outside the group

Usually, on this point, our clients receive only one guideline: if they decide to talk to each other outside the group, they are invited to communicate that to the group itself, in order to facilitate an understanding of the dynamics of their interactions. Therapists, on the other hand, can never cross that boundary and cannot join informal meetings with members, such as drinks, dinners, private parties, or ceremonies like weddings and graduations.

Nonetheless, it is advised to remember that interactions between members outside of a therapy setting can give way to complications. Some clients might expect that the intimacy perceived with others within the group carries outside the group unchanged. However, unlike what happens in the outside world, in the safety of the group setting, interactions happen in their reduced and simplified form and, thanks to the therapist's support and members' high motivation levels, the work of analysis and mediation during sessions is facilitated. Group members also have to learn that group intimacy is a product of a specific relational skill they are in the process of acquiring and that they will be able to employ to make new friends and forge new bonds in the outside world.

An interesting case took place when Lizzy's decision to drop out of group therapy was motivated by conflict, since she did not feel understood by the therapist. In that occasion, Lizzy invited the whole group to dinner, to say goodbye without the therapist. During the course of dinner, Lizzy looked for allies to ferociously criticize the therapist. Thus, the reunion ended in a most unpleasant way for all involved, and during the next session, everyone declared that they would prefer not to find themselves in a similar situation ever again, and for this reason, they had decided not to see each other outside the group.

WhatsApp groups

In the last couple of years, we are witnessing a tendency from members to recreate the group through digital technologies, such as WhatsApp, with the specific aim to keep in touch during the week. In some cases, it was the therapist themselves who created these groups to facilitate the sharing of information regarding changes in time or urgent communications. The fact that group members have at their disposal a digital space in which to pour their thoughts and feelings entails certain risks of which the therapist should be aware. The multiplying of transactions outside the agreed-upon setting during the course of the whole week is certainly an unfavorable matter. Some clients use the WhatsApp group to talk about their nightly crisis, or even to communicate their decision to suspend treatment, saying goodbye to other members. As supervisors of therapists, we have often suggested not to allow the creation of such groups and to confront members about it in case they decided to spontaneously activate these types of interactions. Rather, therapists can fruitfully use WhatsApp's broadcast lists, which allow for a quick and easy manner to send the same message to multiple individual users at the same time, without having to create a group. Only during extraordinary circumstances – such as the lockdown period in Italy caused by the Covid-19 outbreak – we have encouraged the creation of WhatsApp groups, and in any case always with the therapist's participation. The purpose of this was to comfort members during a difficult time characterized by the deep deprivation of social distancing norms, imposed by the government in an effort to safeguard public health. The resulting social experiment was very interesting and all clients involved managed to strengthen their sense of belonging to the group, increasing overall cohesion.

Gina takes advantage of a WhatsApp group created for communications during lockdown leaving long, rambling voice messages without actually attending the next therapy session. In the beginning, members take their time listening to her and comforting her, but after a while, they grow annoyed and decide to discuss this matter during a session. "It's not fair you make us worry about you without giving us the chance to talk stuff through with you" – says Terry – and the others point out to Gina that they have stopped listening to her messages because she has become overwhelming. Thus, the group negotiates new boundaries for the use of WhatsApp: from that moment on, it will be used only when other means of communication are unavailable or for brief communications, for example in case of an unforeseen event preventing a client from attending the next session.

A clinical example of the negotiation of group behavior

Fabrizio (40 years old) joined a group recently. He is annoyed when he sees Rosa (45 years old) being very nonchalant and taking off her shoes to curl up in her armchair and rest her bare feet on the fabric. Giulia (35 years old) comes to the meeting directly from work and is always very hungry, so she often eats a sandwich during the first few minutes of the session. After a few meetings, Fabrizio blurts out:

> What's even happening in this group, you don't have any respect for each other. You (Rosa) take the liberty of taking off your shoes and put your feet on the armchair, and you (Giulia) leave crumbs everywhere. I'd like to know how you, as therapist, can allow all this.

In the beginning Rosa and Giulia get offended and the rest of the group takes their side, defending the "elder" members and rejecting Fabrizio, the newcomer. Then, a particularly stimulating debate takes place regarding which kind of behavior each of them finds adequate or inadequate in that context. Fabrizio tells the group that in his family, they were forbidden to take off their shoes and walk barefoot, and his mother would not allow her children to eat outside meals or sitting on the sofas. He also recounts the punishments and the strictness of his family environment. Rosa and Giulia, at that point, are much more inclined to welcome him, after ironically saying that Fabrizio's fearful mother seemed to have joined the group as well.

A clinical example of the violation of an unwritten norm

Ingrid (55 years old) enters a therapy group following her psychiatrist's advice, who is treating her because of a major depression associated with alcoholism. After six months of therapy, she starts to skip some meetings. Group members try to confront her about it during sessions, fearing a relapse. One night she arrives in a taxi, considerably late, and it is immediately clear to everyone she is drunk and confused. The therapist confronts her among everyone's embarrassment. Ingrid confesses that night she had decided to stop hiding from others: she is just a dirty old drunkard. The group jumps to her aid: a member goes to make her a camomile, another acknowledges her bravery in revealing herself, and another points out she avoided driving and safely called a taxi instead. Everyone says: *we'll talk about everything else during the next meeting, when you're sober. For now, you rest and take care, you aren't clear-headed right now and we don't want to give in to your impulse of being punished by us.*

Conclusions

What we have presented here are a few clear guidelines, but it is important to remember that the rest is up for debate and analysis. For all the reasons we have mentioned, we prefer to limit ourselves to stressing to our clients the importance of their commitment to confidentiality regarding what happens within the group and the composition of the group itself. For what concerns the request to make themselves available to give and receive sincere feedback, to dedicate three final sessions to closure before ending treatment, and to pay the agreed-upon fee also in case of absence, these are presented in the form of an Adult–Adult agreement, in order not to force anyone to join the group out of duty, that is, letting the client's Adapted Child – over-charged of parental rules – decide in their stead.

References

EATA. (2011). *Ethical code*. Retrieved from www.eatanews.org

Tangolo, A. E. (2015). *Psychodynamic psychotherapy with transactional analysis: Theory and narration of a living experience* (A. Iozzelli & K. Jones, Trans.). London: Karnac (Originally published in 2010).

Yalom, I. D., & Leszcz, M. (2005). *The theory and practice of group psychotherapy* (5th ed.). New York: Basic Books (Originally published in 1970).

7

THERAPEUTIC ALLIANCE AND CONTRACTS

The therapeutic alliance is the psychological aspect of the relationship between client and therapist which facilitates collaboration in order to reach the common goal of the treatment. In group, cohesion between members is the climate that allows people to feel part of a whole and participate in the exchanges taking place. Here, the therapeutic alliance implies cohesion because the bond between therapist and client cannot be enough.

Therefore, there is a therapeutic alliance specific to groups which involves cohesion between members and the therapist. The sense of belonging and worth, or, as Yalom defines it (Yalom & Leszcz, 2005), the sense of "we-ness" experienced by the individual members help us better understand this concept.

Cohesion is indeed perceived by each member as a feeling of belonging to a "we," which allows them to maintain a coherent sense of self. According to Schore (2020), this feeling is connected to the right frontal lobe and constitutes the "glue holding together a sense of self" (p. 18). Transposing these considerations from an individual to a group setting, we can say that cohesion contributes to the development, in members, of emotion regulation functions and attachment bonds (as we have already seen in Chapter 4), especially when the group shares deep emotional experiences.

In the beginning, members feel cohesion in the form of support and acceptance by the group. Gradually, this perception goes on to create an interrelation between trust in the group and an increased self-esteem.

If in individual therapy, the therapeutic alliance is determined by insight, transference, and countertransference relations and the sharing of common goals; in group therapy, it is connected to the interactions between members, to the climate within the group, and to the focus on the relationship between the self and others, thus confirming that other members are the main source of change for each client.

According to several studies (Taft, Murphy, Musser, & Remington, 2004; Lorentzen, Sexton, & Høglend, 2004), the creation of a good alliance in the first stage of group therapy may predict a favorable outcome of the treatment.

DOI: 10.4324/9781003215547-8

Contractual alliance

For transactional analysts, the contract is a fundamental tool in building the alliance. Novellino defines it "the conscious counterpart of transference alliance."

The contract is an explicit agreement between therapist and client concerning the therapy goals and the methods that will be adopted in order to reach those goals. Unlike what happens in an individual setting, clients join a group with a goal in mind, previously defined during one-on-one therapy, and with basic knowledge of the working principles of group treatment.

Thus, each client joining a group consented to this experience and signed a document in which all administrative and organizational agreements are made explicit. After having clearly expressed rules and guidelines, the therapist invites each member to discuss these topics with the group. It is interesting from the point of view of analytical work, to observe how people react to requests such as being on time, notifying absences, and paying for the sessions following the agreed-upon methods. Anything can be discussed in group, even the fact that at times each member considers their seat as untouchable by others.

"You came first and took my armchair" says Katy ferociously to a fellow member, "You know that's my seat," and Luca answers back: "Yes, I did it on purpose because I think we all need to change our perspective from time to time." The discussion that follows is rather fruitful: each member is able to express their opinion allowing others to get to know them a little better and verify that the context is safe enough to share deeper parts of themselves.

This stage corresponds to the provisional group imago described by Berne (see Chapter 12), when members depend heavily on the leader, who becomes idealized, and their expectations regarding the group are influenced by their own life stories, and, most of all, by previous experiences in their groups of origin they have had in their lives. The therapist will ask clients to talk spontaneously and honestly, following the rules of peaceful coexistence.

The impulses will have to be expressed verbally and never acted upon. Moreover, the therapist will invite everyone to regularly attend group sessions until the goals made explicit in the contract are reached. As we have mentioned in Chapter 6, confidentiality is the only guideline that is necessary to protect the group: not only the therapist, but all members will have to avoid exposing other members by bringing up any material that has emerged in the course of treatment, outside the group. It is especially this last point we deem necessary to bring into sharp focus.

When the group becomes important for the individual members, it is natural that they wish to share with their loved ones what they have learned in therapy. Nonetheless, it is of paramount importance that they avoid revealing other members' names and identities.

A client's violation of this rule will entail their suspension from group therapy, which will be replaced by individual therapy until the client is able to take responsibility and commit to respecting the group's privacy and boundaries (Moiso, 1998, p. 74).

The next step for each client is sharing the individual contract subscribed with the therapist before joining the group. Some therapists suggest clients do that through drawing or projective games such as guided fantasies. The choice to use creative expression techniques depends mostly on the therapist's style. In any case, it is important that each client share their contract with all members so that the group might support them in their journey. Indeed, the initial exercises and the encouragement to share facilitate the building of group cohesion and strengthen the alliance.

Sharing the individual contract within the group, moreover, allows the client to be able to project themselves in the future and anticipate the emotions they might experience when they finally reach the agreed-upon goals, linking these hopeful and trusting emotions to the anxiety and disorientation which pervaded their past and to their present lives. These are the client's first steps toward a narrative coherence, a slow and gradual acceptance of their own history, which is crucial to understand the mental states underlying their own behaviors, as well as others'.

For subjects suffering from more serious illnesses, formulating a contract within a group before seven or eight pairs of attentive and scrutinizing eyes – taking on the responsibility of working toward difficult goals, as the acquisition of emotion regulation skills and the verbalization of emotions which were acted upon by virtue of being misunderstood – represents a true challenge, and as such should always be highlighted and encouraged.

When a member renders explicit the goals appearing in their contract, the therapist must encourage the group's collaboration, seeking everyone's contribution in order to help the speaker make their goals reachable. For example, if one of the client's goals is to be able to face their fear of other people's judgment and to be more spontaneous and open to intimacy, the therapist might ask the following questions: "Are you willing to share your discomfort in case you receive negative feedback? So that we might better understand your fears?" Or:

> How can we know if you are having trouble since I asked everyone to be willing to give and receive feedback freely? And again: Is there some request you want to make of the group that might help you accept also negative strokes, and prevent you from closing yourself off completely, as you told us you usually do in real life?

Should the therapist notice similarities between the agreed-upon goals of two or more clients? It is important that they encourage these clients to talk about what it feels like to see other people living with their same afflictions but also the same hopes, actively promoting, already in this stage, interactions between group members, as well as focusing on the reciprocal and collaborative nature of psychotherapy.

According to Yalom, individuals whose needs share similarities with other members tend to strengthen group cohesion (Yalom & Leszcz, 2005).

Alliance between ruptures and resolutions

We have said that the alliance is connected to group cohesion, that is, the appeal the group has on its members and the multiple collaborative bonds which develop between members during the group process, on both a cognitive and emotional level.

Empathy, self-disclosure, trust, and acceptance are fundamental elements which characterize the relational alliance. This builds gradually from an adapted group imago, through an operative group imago, and arrives at a secondarily adjusted group imago (we will explore this further in Chapter 12). It is a slow and complex process, more dynamic than static, which involves several ruptures and resolutions, and which begins, as we have seen earlier, from as early as the contractual stage.

The alliance must not be confused with the acceptance and understanding between members, but it is connected to these factors through an interdependent relation (Yalom & Leszcz, 2005). A client joins the group for the first time and interprets the hostility they perceive from others as a sign that the group is not a safe space; later, however, when their sense of belonging will have developed, they will be able to face conflicts and learn from affectionate interactions. Overcoming conflict dynamics gives back to each member a sense of belonging to a community in which all parts of themselves are accepted and where it is safe to share their thoughts. A coherent group enjoys a higher degree of intimacy between its members and, therefore, conflicts emerge openly.

When the alliance between members and therapist, or between members themselves, ruptures, collaboration within the group stops and the group climate becomes aggressive: sometimes that aggression is expressed openly; other times, it is hidden behind walls of silence. Games prevail, and all subjects, including the therapist, take on the roles of the Drama Triangle (Karpman, 1968): some play the role of the Victim, some play the role of the Persecutor, and some play the role of the Rescuer. Then, there is the Bystander (Clarkson, 1987), who closes off in silence and does not dare to speak.

These are delicate moments, but if the therapist is able to deal with this relational impasse, the group alliance might come out of it considerably stronger. In such cases, everything hinges on how the therapist faces the members' resistance to change within group dynamics.

If the therapist is too rigid and lacks the necessary flexibility to understand the members' individual needs and to accommodate them within the treatment, or if they collude with the client's anger because of their scarce tolerance to conflict or a strong need for approval, it will be more difficult for the group to resolve any rupture and create a narrative in which conflicts make sense. Containing conflict between members without interrupting, it is a job that well-rounded therapists must be prepared to undertake. The subjects involved in conflict need a space in which to elaborate it, in order to take responsibility for their words and build a solid foundation for a productive use of tolerance. If, outside the group, within social environments, conflicts often lead to permanent ruptures in relationships, within the group, tolerating discomfort leads instead to the discovery of a freedom that is respectful of differences. At the basis of these, cycles of rupture and resolution, however, must lay the condition of cohesion.

Only in a coherent group, everyone understands the importance they hold in each other's eyes, and the atmosphere is filled by a strong sense of mutual loyalty; it is possible to derive benefit from conflict.

Thus, tolerance wards off the risk of becoming a mere adaptation to the needs of others, or a laxity toward the fastidious turmoil which disrupts the circle, and instead becomes an impulse fueled by critical thought which proceeds toward an understanding of what happens in the external as well as in the internal reality.

Alba is a middle-aged woman who started group therapy six months ago. At 15 years old, she was abused by an older cousin 10 years her senior and this violence "has left its mark on her," words she often repeats in individual therapy. Daughter of a depressed mother, she has never dared to talk to anyone about her trauma; at the time of the incident, in fact, she was taking care of her mother and her disabled brother – three years older than her – who, at the time, had been hospitalized for serious health concerns related to his disability. She has a good relationship with her husband, their bond is full of trust and they enjoy spending time together doing all kinds of activities, except sex. Alba's body kept count of all wounds inflicted to her. Some sort of indelible trace which prevents her from feeling pleasure from penetration.

One night, Mery, another group member the same age as Alba, recounts her childhood with a psychotic mother, whose rather bizarre behaviors used to be a source of deep shame for Mery in front of friends and relatives. It was only as an Adult that Mery then discovered from her dad that her mother had been raped by a neighbor at a young age. Alba listens to the whole thing frowning, an expression of anger and pain on her face, fists clenched. Toward the end of the session, the therapist, worried about her, asks her how she feels and what kind of emotion she is ending the session with. Alba mutters something under her breath such as "all good" and keeps looking at the clock as if expecting the school bell's ring in order to escape the anxiety of a test. The following day, Alba phones her therapist to communicate her intention of leaving the group. The tone of her voice is final, as if to say that nothing will convince her otherwise. During the individual session which Alba accepted to have at the insistence of the therapist, to process together this sudden decision, the client expresses her furious anger toward the therapist, guilty, in her eyes, to have asked the question at the end of the session in order to force her to talk in front of everyone about her trauma.

There are moments during the therapeutic process, and the therapist knows it well, in which responding to a client's anger with rationalizations or explanations of their reasons is useless or even counter-productive. There are times when silence is the best container for an enormous amount of pain. There are times when silence speaks:

> Yes, I know you felt raped all over again and this time by me, you perceived me as someone who wanted to penetrate your inner world and direct your words. You have the right to access all this even if my intent was only to know how you felt.

Listening lends strength to therapy. And while they listen, a part of the therapist really feels "bad"; *after all*, they ask themselves, *why ask such a stupid question moments before the end of the session*? This is the projective transference mentioned by Hargaden and Sills (2002): the client's Child, angry and full of shame, is projected onto the therapist because Alba cannot bear to experience it. The fear of being penetrated has always overcome Alba, forcing her to put her life on a path that did not belong to her. Her job as a nurse allows her to take care of others and not feel vulnerable. She had already built a fortress around her a long time before that she was abused. She had learned how to be a nurse during her childhood, when she would try to fix her mother's spiritual wounds, by trying to make her laugh, or making herself invisible in her eyes in order not to cause any problems: she had become a very good mum to her mother and brother.

That outburst served as an important turning point for Alba: it allowed her to recognize, for the first time in her life, a maternal figure able to contain her emotional intensity without falling to pieces. Together therapist and client contributed to the integration of Alba's dissociated parts, those vulnerable parts of her who had been reactivated in group and in the here-and-now of the therapeutic process in pursuit of a new kind of balance.

Alba, reexperiencing that terrible traumatic event, had felt the need to create a new rupture, this time in her alliance with the group. Her life had been interrupted by the abuse and now she had interrupted her experience of the group, perceived as abusing toward her. After three months of processing her traumas in individual therapy, Alba decided to rejoin the group.

During those three months, she had built a new alliance with the therapist. As she commented afterward, she started trusting her only after that episode, which allowed her to finally feel like a daughter. After her return, her relationship with the others was subject to profound changes: her script belief telling her that "others can hurt me again if I show any vulnerability" lost considerable power, and she gradually started to experience a much more spontaneous way of dealing with conflict, taking responsibility for her pain and at the same time allowing others to take care of her. Alba left the group after three years of intense work which ended up strengthening the boundaries between her ego states as well as her Adult. The internal dialogue between a Rescuer Parent and a Victim Child gave way to an efficient communication between a Nurturing Parent and a Child who has overcome shame and has become capable of asking for attention and care from the outside world. However, Alba's fellow group members also grew after seeing her leave the group and then come back three months later. During this time, Mery was also able to process her guilt with regard to Alba, who she had perceived as a too-fragile mother – much like her real mother – whom she had hurt and "cast out" from the group. Everyone learned that relationships can fall apart, but ruptures may give way to constructive resolutions through the creation of a space in which to process and explore possible ways to contribute to the conflict and its resolution.

Conclusions

Guilt is always present when there is a rupture in the group alliance. The game of "Courtroom" prevails over the possibility of a shared Adult thought, as we have seen in the case of Alba and Mery. "It's my fault," "it's always my fault," "it's all your fault," "it's always so and so's fault." Guilt, when maladaptive, is accompanied by intense shame, as Weiss reminds us (Weiss, 1993). It stems from traumatic experiences in attachment relationships during childhood.

Trapped in shame and guilt, clients tend to close off or project an emotional intensity too difficult to contain on the therapist or their fellow members. Closure or projection are indeed dissociative modes that traumatized people use to cope with intra-psychic conflicts. For this reason, ruptures are important and delicate moments: they shake the group's cohesion but they possess a great therapeutic value. They allow to reexperience on an implicit level the first autobiographical memories of the script protocols, in order to explore affections and dissociated or repressed emotions through stimuli offered by other members. Unconscious dissociated shame is experienced once again, but this time it is shared intersubjectively through the preverbal emotional resonance of the right brain. The synchronization of the right brains amplifies the intensity of this experience, allowing unconscious affections to enter both individual's and group's awareness, thus regulating them interactively (Schore, 2020).

We can use the metaphor of kintsugi in order to describe the cycles of ruptures and resolutions which characterize the alliance. When a bowl, a precious vase, or a teapot fall down, breaking to pieces, with this Japanese technique, it is possible not only to reassemble the broken pottery item but even embellish it using melted iron or lacquer mixed with powdered gold, in order to highlight the new cracks. Thanks to the new metal-enhanced ramifications, each item becomes unique and irreplaceable.

When two or more people within a group share an intense emotional experience, no matter the nature of the emotion, old wounds are fixed and the container/group's ramifications take on new shapes, enhancing and restoring each client's uniqueness.

References

Clarkson, P. (1987). The Bystander role. *Transactional Analysis Journal*, *17*(3), 82–87. doi:10.1177/036215378701700305

Hargaden, H., & Sills, C. (2002). *Transactional analysis: A relational perspective*. New York: Brunner-Routledge.

Karpman, S. (1968). Fairy tales and script drama analysis. *Transactional Analysis Bulletin*, *7*(26), 39–43.

Lorentzen, S., Sexton, H. C., & Høglend, P. (2004). Therapeutic alliance, cohesion and outcome in a long-term analytic group: A preliminary study. *Nordic Journal of Psychiatry*, *58*(1), 33–40. doi:10.1080/08039480310000770

Moiso, C. (1998). Il setting in psicoterapia di gruppo. In M. Novellino (Ed.), *L'approccio clinico dell'Analisi Transazionale*. Milano: Franco Angeli.

Novellino, M. (1998). *L'approccio clinico dell'analisi transazionale*. Milano: Franco Angeli.

Schore, N. A. (2020). Forging connections in group psychotherapy through right brain-to-right brain emotional communications. Part 1: Theoretical models of right brain therapeutic action. Part 2: Clinical case analyses of group right brain regressive enactments. *International Journal of Group Psychotherapy*, *70*(1), 29–88. doi:10.1080/00207284.2019.1682460

Taft, C. T., Murphy, C. M., Musser, P. H., & Remington, N. A. (2004). Personality, Interpersonal, and motivational predictors of the working alliance in group cognitive-behavioral therapy for partner violent men. *Journal of Consulting and Clinical Psychology*, *72*(2), 349–354. doi:10.1037/0022-006X.72.2.349

Weiss, J. (1993). *How psychotherapy works: Process and technique*. New York: Guilford Press.

Yalom, I. D., & Leszcz, M. (2005). *The theory and practice of group psychotherapy* (5th ed.). New York: Basic Books (Originally published in 1970).

8

DECONTAMINATION WORK IN A GROUP SETTING

What is contamination?

In transactional analysis, doing decontamination work means freeing the Adult ego state from certain beliefs that were introjected, respectively, by the Parent ego state, in the shape of generalizations and prejudices, and by the Child ego state, in the shape of phobias and illusions. In *Transactional Analysis in Psychotherapy*, Berne wrote that "contamination is best illustrated by certain types of prejudice on the one hand [Parent contaminating the Adult], and by delusions on the other [Child contaminating the Adult]" (Berne, 1961, p. 47) In *What Do You Say After Hello?* (Berne, 1972, p. 155), he also wrote that contaminations of the Child are "illusions." Clarkson (1992, p. 20) argues that

> the concept of contamination describes the way in which effective Adult functioning is impeded by the scripting process. Contamination can occur when Parent ego states intrude upon the Adult (e.g. *prejudices*) or when the Child ego states intrude upon the Adult (e.g. *phobias*).

When applied to the structural model of the ego states, the concept of contamination explains how a person, while interacting with others and themselves, loses rationality and adherence to the here-and-now in reality testing. So, for example, when a client, at the beginning of therapy, referring to the efficacy of the treatment, says: "I don't believe in these things," we can postulate that their Adult ego state is not entirely clear-headed. If we analyze the content of such a sentence, we will find the presence of implicit assumptions: the conviction that one must "believe" in a method or theory as if it was a faith, the fear of psychological dependence from a mind which could influence their own, and perhaps the echo of their mother's words, who used to tell them "not to accept candies from strangers" or "not to talk to strangers about what happens in the house" because "you shouldn't wash your dirty linen in public."

DOI: 10.4324/9781003215547-9

Cavallero (1998, p. 103) wrote that

> one of the reasons leading to or preserving contamination is to be found in the economical principle of minimal effort, according to which a big part of our life is made easier to manage through a series of automatisms, beliefs, habits, assumptions, or references to obsolete experiences.

Starting treatment

At the beginning of a treatment, it is very important to explore with our clients their contaminated beliefs. This helps them envision with more clarity the first goals of therapy: freeing the Adult ego state and restoring its power and control over their person.

Another example of contamination may be found in the guilt experienced by some clients in relation to their depression. This belief expresses itself in statements such as "I am not capable of being in the world," "After all, it is my fault if I feel bad because I'm lazy and indolent, as my father used to say," and "I don't make enough of an effort."

In these cases, we are facing a double contamination. On the one hand, the Parent contaminates the Adult with prejudices such as "If you try hard enough you will be able to overcome all obstacles" and "Where there is a will there is a way." On the other hand, the Child needs to believe in the illusion that if they try harder they will be able to reach any kind of goal.

Contaminations in group

In response to the invitation to join a therapy group, some clients might activate specific defenses or resistances, expressed by such prejudices as "Groups are dangerous," "Others are always judgmental," and "Relationships are hornets' nests and I will end up being ignored and ridiculed because my problems don't matter in the eyes of others." For others, the contaminating agent is the illusion to find within the group the love they lacked in life: when these clients ask us therapists if there exists a possibility of falling in love with a group member, their question somehow echoes what Berne (1961) defined as the illusion of Santa Claus, Prince charming or the damsel in distress.

As therapists, we can consider these statements as script beliefs and treat them as themes pointing out to a confusion of the Child ego state. However, it is useful to treat such statements from the very beginning as elements of an apparently "Adult" but actually contaminated discourse, that is constrained by the insurgence of archaic influences and introjections.

Decontamination techniques

Group therapy is the setting of choice for the main technique of intervention on contamination, that is, confrontation. Chapters 10 and 11 will include a specific

73

section on this mode of intervention. For the moment, it is enough to reiterate the importance of working strategically with clients to clear the space where the Adult should be. This is a necessary condition to the strengthening of the therapeutic alliance and the fostering, in clients, of the awareness which allows them to move forward with their treatment and become, in time, their own co-therapist, as well as other members'.

Thus, for example, the belief expressed by a group member of not being able to trust anyone outside their family may easily be confronted by other members. Someone might object that, often, a betrayal of trust comes precisely from the family folds and might proceed to tell specific episodes disproving such a generalization.

Voicing prejudices and generalizations often contributes to make apparent their most ridiculous features: thus, the voicing of statements which have been resonating in their head since childhood might lead clients to question the system of reference from which the statements come from and start distancing themselves from them. At the same time, it is especially by explaining the reasons behind their illusions and phobias to someone else that it is possible for the clients to uncover the fundamental irrationality of their beliefs.

The strategic cognitive phase to strengthen the Adult

"Decontamination means that where the patient's reactions, feelings, or viewpoints are adulterated or distorted, the situation will be rectified by a process analogous to that of anatomical dissection" (Berne, 1966, p. 213).

During this strategic phase of the therapy, the group works as a space for exchange and learning which focuses on cognitive work. This is an aspect of the group setting which makes TA group therapy the most of cognitive among the various types of psychodynamic therapy.

At the third stage in the evolution of a group (see Chapter 11) this level of exchange dominates transactions and adds to therapeutic process with respect to the individual setting. Indeed, the group may facilitate the development of cognitive dissonance in the client through a peer-to-peer confrontation in which the therapist remains neutral, inviting the client themselves to reflect on the social impact of their own messages. The aim is to "maintain sufficient pressure for the dissonance to be resolved by the client rejecting the old belief, accepting the compelling logic of the argument and developing a new belief" (Widdowson, 2015, p. 114).

A clinical example

The aim of this therapeutic intervention, continues Widdowson, is "assisting a client and identifying her own vicious cycles" because "once your client can recognize her own vicious cycles, you can engage her in a discussion about how she can interrupt these patterns" (Widdowson, 2015, p. 119).

The following is an excerpt of group therapy in which a depressed client, Sara, complains, and the group reacts to this transactional stimulus.

SARA: [Sighing deeply] I keep feeling unwell, this is not working, not meds nor the group, I'm desperate . . .

SONIA: You've been complaining for several months without doing anything to change things.

SARA: You mean it's my fault if I feel like this? You sound like my mother: always criticizing me.

ALESSIO: Sara, maybe you should take Sonia's words as an invite to take charge of your situation, and not just complain.

LUIGI: But now it sounds like everyone is attacking Sara.

SARA: Thanks, Luigi. You're the only one on my side. I feel like you're there for me.

DEBORA: Sara, it seems we can't help you in any way, maybe we feel a little frustrated because we've been trying for months.

THERAPIST: Should we take a moment to think about what's happening between us right now?

SARA: Alright.

> Sonia, Alessio, Debora, and Luigi agree.
>
> The therapist draws Sara's ego states on the board and asks the group: Which ego state was Sara speaking from?

DEBORA: A complaining Child.

SONIA: I felt like it was a Critical Parent who wanted to take Sara away from the group by criticizing everyone and everything and saying "It's not working."

ALESSIO: I was also bothered by the criticism.

LUIGI: Well, it's understandable since she doesn't feel any better.

THERAPIST: See, Sara, you have a great need to be understood and to feel like everyone is on your side, but that rarely happens. Why do you think?

SARA: Of course, I understand that the others don't like the Critical Parent, and that listening to the complaining Child gets tired and boring.

THERAPIST: Can you find other ways to ask for closeness?

SARA: So, it's been another difficult week for me and sometimes I feel desperate. I still can't get back on my feet.

SONIA: I feel like I should respect your struggle, which is mine too. The anxiety is still very much here.

For Sara, becoming aware of the impact of her words on the others was fundamental. Seeing the trap in which she was about to fall into was a stimulus to experiment with other ways to ask for attention. Sara's complaint at the beginning of this excerpt could have pushed the therapist to lead the work in different directions. Their choice, however, was to let Sara interact with other members. This way, first, she acquired a greater awareness of what was happening, and later, invited by the therapist themselves, she was able to start experimenting with a different way to express her despondency and cry for help.

The use of the Drama Triangle in group psychotherapy for clients with personality disorders

Some transactional analysis models employing a simplified illustration of ego states, games, and transactions are especially helpful to activate clients and increase their involvement in the therapeutic process and analysis.

Steve Karpman's Drama Triangle model is also used in settings and approaches which differ considerably from ours. In a famous paper from 1968, later published in the book *A Game Free Life* (2014), Karpman (1968) proposes a model in which people enter a relational game assuming at times the role of Victim, Rescuer, and Persecutor, trapping themselves into unhappy relationship schemes. In this dynamic, at some point, there comes a shift which Eric Berne defines as typical of psychological games, in which, for example, a Rescuer, tired of putting considerable effort into saving a complaining Victim, switches to the role of Persecutor, concluding that "in the end, you asked for it and you deserve the failure in which you find yourself into." By the same logic, a Victim may assume the role of Persecutor, causing their Rescuer to become a Victim. These renowned analysis models of unhappy interpersonal dynamics are especially useful when doing decontamination work in a group, because they help clients understanding what happens between people and encourage them to look for different modes of behavior.

In that regard, some Italian studies (Fassone, Ivaldi, & Rocchi, 2003; Fassone, Ivaldi, Mantione, & Rocchi, 2004) found that drop-out rates in the treatment model integrating individual and group therapy for clients suffering from personality disorders, was lower than those related to clients undergoing individual treatment. Among the descriptive and therapeutic tools employed by researchers during group treatment, Karpman's Drama Triangle (Fassone et al., 2004) proved to be an interactive scheme particularly useful to improve awareness in the here-and-now of their own dysfunctional relational models, as well as others'. In a group setting, the Drama Triangle is employed since the very beginning of treatment: in the contractual stage, the therapist explains to the group what this tool is and how it can be used during sessions by members and therapist alike. For example, if, in making their contract explicit, a member expresses their need to learn how to regulate their anger in order to have more constructive interactions with others, it will be useful for them to receive information from the therapist on how the Drama Triangle may be used in the therapeutic process to contain their hostility and avoid its redirection toward other members and therapist. In this case, the therapeutic operation of explanation aims to encourage members' active participation and collaboration, promoting a culture of responsibility within the group. In the next stages of the group process, they will be able to independently experience this interactive scheme when understanding and giving meaning to the activation of one of the dramatic roles. The games played in group and described through the Drama Triangle allow clients to process the script experiences thanks to everyone's willingness to give and receive feedback, enhancing reflective thinking and thus empowering the members' Adult ego state. Fassone et al. (2004) remark that it is necessary for therapists to understand which role of the Triangle they tend to take on more frequently, in order to avoid possible collusions with members. In relation to clients with a troubled past and suffering from personality disorders, who are trapped into the role of Victim or Persecutor, for example, the therapist is often led to play the role of the Rescuer.

Understanding their own elements of countertransference allows the therapist to position themselves outside of the Drama Triangle, in order to facilitate a conscious reading of what happens in the here-and-now of the group experience.

We deem it relevant to note that, in Fassone and colleagues' study, the Drama Triangle proved itself to be a useful tool to revisit the here-and-now client-to-client and client-to-therapist interactions happening in group therapy. However, in that case, researchers took a cognitive-evolutionary approach, even if they relied on TA tools.

Therefore, it is important to understand the differences between a cognitive-evolutionary and a transactional analysis approach to group therapy.

According to cognitivist psychotherapists, a therapist "should not collude with the patient's need to make a Rescuer out of them" (Fassone et al., 2004, p. 112). Instead, they should keep themselves out of games in order to better help clients alter their interpersonal distortions. Berne, too, believes that the therapist's duty is to observe their clients' script in action from the sidelines, as if they were sitting in the audience, about to assist to "an ongoing drama that is actually taking place right now, divided into scenes and acts" (Berne, 1972, p. 57). Indeed, according to him, it would be a countertransference mistake on the therapist's part, to let themselves be involved in the clients' games (Berne, 1964).

However, many scholars in the TA field, as we shall see in Chapter 13, have distanced themselves from this unilateral perception of games in which clients are the only one playing, turning instead to a bidirectional conception, in which games are played by everyone, therapist and clients alike (Stuthridge, 2015; Cornell Hargaden, & Allen, 2005; Hargaden & Sills, 2002). In the treatment of clients suffering from personality disorders, countertransference, which is often induced in the form of enactment (the therapist identifies with the elements which the client, unable to bear seeing in themselves, projects onto them) becomes, according to these scholars, a crucial element for the understanding of the unconscious communication happening between clients and therapist within a intersubjective dynamic.

Conclusions

The aim of decontamination is thus to widen the space for the Adult within the client. This will help them in improving their decision-making processes as well as in understanding their symptoms and in becoming aware that said symptoms might disappear or be kept under control, thus becoming more easily bearable and curable.

> So, for example, often in group, we might hear a client who, talking about their symptoms of anxiety, says something like: "I'm here thanks to panic attacks, and I was forced to put a stop to a frenetic life which was spinning out of control as fast a manic merry-go-round," as stated by Carmen in a moment of awareness, while she welcomed in the group a new person who introduced herself as suffering from a particularly crippling anxiety disorder.

In another group, Sabine, confronting Sonia about her obsessive-compulsive disorder (OCD) symptoms, revealed that her relationship with the group was particularly useful to her in understanding the origin of her need for control.

Clarkson (1992, p. 105) argued that "the client's energy increases in the here-and-now as it is withdrawn from involvement with the 'there-and-then,' away from adaptive script fixations and towards the service of the biological organism in its present environment with the present wants and needs."

Decontamination is thus useful to stabilize the Adult ego state, to allow the client to take back control of their behavior, increasing medication compliance (if necessary), and stimulating the client to take steps toward protection and constructive collaboration with the group.

For many clients, reaching a relative behavioral stability and increasing self-awareness leads to an improvement in their mental health, which is already quite a result. So, for example, for some clients sharing with the group their own Parent-contaminated beliefs, especially with regard to their affective and sexual choices, can be rather important. Indeed, in doing so, they are able to indirectly extrapolate a permission to be okay if their choice of sexual partners fails be understood or shared by the familial system of origin. Thus, the group proves itself quite useful in battling internalized homophobia, lesbophobia, biphobia, and transphobia in both cis-heterosexual clients and otherwise, and in opening their minds to a wider variety of options for love and happiness. The group provides opportunities for comparison with systems of reference that are more open and modern than the client's introjected ones also with regard to important choices in work and education. Thus, for example, many clients might feel inadequate to make decisions regarding a job change, feeling guilty for rejecting a job they do not love because

"I am passing up a once-in-a-lifetime opportunity" or because "you don't leave a steady job" (beliefs of a typical Italian parent, which are still a major influence on younger generations).

When the mind opens up and the client receives from the group a message such as

> Why take into account your father's opinion when he is a farmer who has a very different experience of the world? Instead, why don't you open up to us who are living in the world at the same time as you, and can understand that in this day and age, job changes and instability are the norm?

the answer might be an insight: "It's true! I'm looking for safety in a person who can't give it to me because his experience of the world is 30 or more years old."

At this stage, even if change has not yet taken root, the relief from pain and isolation usually increases the client's willingness to move forward toward greater goals, in order to fill their life with more joy, success, and serenity.

References

Berne, E. (1961). *Transactional analysis in psychotherapy: A systematic individual and social psychiatry*. New York: Grove Press.

Berne, E. (1964). *Games people play: The psychology of human relationships*. New York: Grove Press.

Berne, E. (1966). *Principles of group treatment*. Oxford: Oxford University Press.

Berne, E. (1972). *What do you say after you say hello?: The psychology of human destiny*. New York: Bantam Books.

Cavallero, G. (1998). La decontaminazione. In M. Novellino (Ed.), *L'approccio clinico all'analisi transazionale*. Milano: Franco Angeli.

Clarkson, P. (1992). *Transactional analysis psychotherapy, an integrated approach*. London and New York: Routledge.

Cornell, W. F., Hargaden, H., & Allen, J. R. (Eds.). (2005). *From transactions to relations: The emergence of a relational tradition in transactional analysis*. Chadlington, Oxfordshire: Haddon Press.

Fassone, G., Ivaldi, A., Mantione, G., & Rocchi, M. (2004). Valutazione degli esiti di un trattamento cognitivo-evoluzionista integrato (individuale-gruppo) per pazienti con disturbi di personalità e/o comorbilità in asse I/II: Uno studio seminaturalistico controllato. *Cognitivismo Clinico, 1*(2), 124–138. Retrieved from www.antonellaivaldi. it/files/3-Fassone-Ivaldicogn.-clin.pdf

Fassone, G., Ivaldi, A., & Rocchi, M. (2003). Riduzione del drop-out nei pazienti con disturbi gravi di personalità: Risultati preliminari di un modello di psicoterapia cognitivo-comportamentale integrata, individuale e di gruppo. *Rivista di Psichiatria, 38*, 241–246.

Hargaden, H., & Sills, C. (2002). *Transactional analysis: A relational perspective*. New York: Brunner-Routledge.

Karpman, S. (1968). Fairy tales and script drama analysis. *Transactional Analysis Bulletin, 7*(26), 39–43.

Karpman, S. (2014). *A game free life: The definitive book on the drama triangle and compassion triangle*. San Francisco, CA: Drama Triangle Publications.

Stuthridge, J. (2015). All the world's a stage: Games, enactment, and countertransference. *Transactional Analysis Journal, 45*(2), 104–116. doi:10.1177/0362153715581174

Widdowson, M. (2015). *Transactional analysis for depression: A step-by-step treatment manual* (1st ed.). London and New York: Routledge. doi:10.4324/9781315746630

9

DECONFUSION WORK IN
A GROUP SETTING

The concepts of script, confusion, and deconfusion

Deconfusion is a term that in transactional analysis defines the deepest psychotherapeutic work aimed at altering the psychical structures and emotional balances sustaining the script.

The script is an intra-psychic safety system which structures the sense of continuity of the self, and provides each individual with a sense of stable identity thanks to which they can say: "I'm the kind of person who," "This always happens to me," "People can always be expected to," and "In the end, life is mostly." Therefore, the term "script" is here understood as the totality of beliefs held by human beings about themselves, their relationship with others, and, in general, the filter through which they interpret their lives. This matrix of beliefs was built in time through an intersubjective and interpersonal process of construction of the self, and it is deeply rooted in emotional and physical systems that predate knowledge and procedural memory. The foundations of the psychological script are laid before birth, during pregnancy. In the biochemical exchange happening in the sea of amniotic liquid – in the loving or anxious warmth of someone else's body – emotions are passed on to the yet-unborn child through the umbilical cord, together with the substances nourishing them. Even after we are born, our skin, which contains and delimits our mind and body, constitutes a boundary, a limit, a strong protection, but, at the same time, a permeable one. Through our skin, we feel strokes, warmth and cold, hugs and slaps, and pleasure and pain, and we start building our relationship with the outside world.

The script, containing the matrix of how we exist in the world, is developed during the first years of a newborn's life, and it is precisely in the Child ego state that we can find its historic origin and the inner dialogue which lay the foundations of our relationship with the self, the primary object of love, and life. The kind of thought behind script decisions is the same intuitive, pre-logical one at the basis of the primary defenses the child uses to survive infancy. However, as expected, this kind of thought proves itself inadequate to guide us through the entirety of our lives. It is confusing, linked to archaic emotions and automatic modes of behavior.

DOI: 10.4324/9781003215547-10

Analyzing the script means developing an awareness of the decisions jointly brought about by the fixation of the archaic needs of the Child and an introjected phantasmic Parent. This intra-psychic pair maintains a solid "loyalty pact" that is difficult to disrupt in adult life.

Ray Little, winner of the Eric Berne Memorial Award 2019, in his important 2006 article "Ego State Relation Units and Resistance to Change," rebuilds the foundations of TA theory as linked to its psychoanalytic matrix:

> the Child is the archaic aspect of the ego, fixated at a previous point in history in response to an inadequately met relational need. For Berne [1961], "The Child is a warped ego state which has become fixated and has changed the direction of the whole subsequent portion of the continuum" (p. 39). The Parent, on the other hand, is the introjected aspect of an other, defensively identified with by the ego.
>
> Blackstone (1993) has previously written on the integration of transactional analysis with object relations. She suggested that the P_1 ego state is analogous to the object in object relations theory and that C_1 is analogous to the self. Therefore, when object relations theorists refer to the object, in transactional analysis we can think in terms of the Parent ego state in the conceptual model. Likewise, when they speak of the self, we can equate it with the Child ego state.
>
> (Little, 2006, p. 8)

Little calls "relational units" the different Parent–Child pairs, and explains how difficult it is to intervene on such a profound level when the client emotionally regards change as a threat to the basic safety this pair represents.

Script analysis

Analyzing the script means developing an awareness of the reasons behind the way we relate to others and the world. It means giving words and meaning to the feeling of sadness and unfathomable emptiness which at times overcome us, to our unreasonable fears or irritability, to the anxiety and tension stored in our neck and shoulders, to the sexual restlessness or the compulsions pushing us toward food or substances, and to the apparently inexplicable anguish we feel the need to soothe in order to sleep, rest, and shut down. Analyzing the script means giving meaning to the bizarre or twisted ways we seek love and success and to our efforts to leave a mark on the world. It means giving a voice to the body, to primary emotions, and to the archaic needs guiding – often irrationally – our most important choices.

This analysis constitutes the first, needed, step in order to solve the puzzle of our archaic decisions, and be able to put together a new, more reasonable design, one more functional to our goals, freer from emotions and beliefs developed in our formative environment: ultimately, freer from our parents and their expectations of us, and freer from the limits of our time and cultural environment.

The key to therapy and its greatest personal and social benefit lie in providing us with a wider range of options at our disposal. The deep psychotherapy we call "script analysis" grants us more freedom, making us less conditioned by the past and more capable to participate in the planning and co-creative building of the world.

Analyzing, treating, or changing the script in a group setting

This is the same direction taken by transactional analysis group therapy: a therapy of the depths, aimed at increasing a person's awareness of how their script works, and their ability to analyze their own behavior and recurring emotions, understand themselves, and take responsibility in determining a positive or negative outcome of events.

Carlo Moiso wrote that

> the aim of transactional analytical therapy is to lead the patient to be able to energize their neopsychic structure – that is, the Adult ego state, – so as to allow them to conduct an accurate reality test, to deal as best as they can with their emotional-affective life, to elaborate principles and values that are the building blocks of impulse control.
>
> (My translation, in Novellino, 1998, p. 70)

Berne (1966, p. 269) wrote that when the clinical work gets deeper, "the therapist is working backward from the phenomena to their origin, from the phenotype to the genotype." The "genotypes" we work with are existential positions and script protocols, which Berne also talked about in the interesting Chapter 11 of his already mentioned 1966 publication.

The process that goes beyond the reactivation of the Adult (decontamination) he calls "clarification" (1966, p. 213) and subsequently he alludes to it by writing that "the analytic deconfusion of the Child is undertaken" (p. 215), referring, in this case, to the process of imago transformation toward healing.

Indeed, group therapy allows a deep emotional experience of implicit relational learning, which leads to a redecision of one's own place in the world and one's idea of self by seeing oneself mirrored in the therapist and fellow group members in a new way.

In group, learning and emotional literacy are indeed concrete experiences: here, members learn how to communicate their thoughts and feelings, how to listen to others' emotions, and how to interact without hurting each other. But they also learn how to fix the emotional wounds they inflict on and receive from others, how to deal with envy and jealousy without destroying themselves or others, and how to relate to unrequited love and other more upsetting emotions. They learn how to face shame and boundaries: essentially, they learn how to be people among people, human beings among human beings.

In group, learning happens both explicitly, through communication, and implicitly, through imitation, mirroring, emotional activation, and the empowerment that comes from having options.

The essential therapeutic steps for the client are as follows:

1   Reexperiencing the past emotional group experiences lived in the family of origin or in the first social learning environment (activation of the preconceived and provisional imago, according to Berne, Clarkson and Tudor).
2   Developing an awareness of script decisions made in order to deal with primary emotions (phase of the adapted imago and the most conflict-fraught experiences).
3   Charting a new course of development for the self by relearning how to interact with others (phase of the secondarily adjusted group imago).
4   Fluctuating – by retracing the steps of the development of the self in group – between resorting to reassuring script defense mechanisms to face all relational events, and curiously experimenting with different models, encouraged by the therapist and fellow members (phase of the operative imago and games).
5   Becoming aware of the new learning processes and of the possibility to extend the new models outside of therapy (phase of the clarified group imago).

Deconfusion work in group

The way the group works on such deep aspects of personality favors the analysis of transference processes. Transference processes happens spontaneously when a client joins a group and, as a consequence, the regression to the Child ego state happens without the therapist's intervention.

The therapist's attention focuses first and foremost on observing how each person joining the group relates to the others, how they try to be accepted and included in the relationship system, and how their behavior manifests and evolves progressively.

In Chapter 12, focused on group imago, we shall see how we can use Berne's model to follow the evolution of the mental representations each member produces with respect to their sense of belonging to the group. We know such representations correspond with what Luborsky and Crits-Christoph (1990) call the Core Conflictual Relationship Theme and thus we can employ the analyses of narrative relational units to analyze the deep change in these representations. In the CCRT model, we can analyze specific narrative relational units and identify in them the primary needs of the self (Wishes), the representation of the object's response (Response of the Other, RO, meaning the other's response to those needs) and, subsequently, the reactions of the self to these responses (Response of the self, RS). Needs, or Wishes, correspond to the C_1 described in transactional analysis, the RO to the P_1, and the RS to the A_1's decisions. In this sequence, we can find the construction of script decisions.

A clinical example

Lisa seeks treatment at the age of 40 years because she fell in unrequited love with a female friend. The revelation of this infatuation and the declaration of her feelings to her friend filled her with surprise and shame. Lisa had never fallen in love before, nor had she had any sexual or romantic relationship.

She lives alone and works with her parents in a small restaurant where she is allowed to hide in the kitchen and avoid any contact with customers. Lisa was a very shy girl, particularly inhibited since she started suffering from epilepsy at the age of six years. Her health issues and introverted nature are, according to her, the reason why she has lived in hiding up until now, as if all her life she had taken "back roads" so as not to be seen. Lisa is suggested group therapy in order to face the shame she feels at being herself and be assisted in a coming out process with the aim of opening up to a romantic life.

Lisa manifests among her *Wishes* her need for contact and intimacy. However, she has introjected rejection as *Response of the other*. Thus, she reacts by abandoning her pursuit for affection and making herself passive, defeatist, and quiet. The decision to seek treatment is made on the heels of the intensification of her desire and the impossibility to sedate the pain stemming from rejection.

In group, Lisa learns how to manifest her desires and needs, as well as seek a healthy way to satisfy them. She learns how to openly frequent gay-friendly environments, where she can look for a partner more easily and feel comfortable enough.

> In my dreams, the group is always there. I'm in the group therapy room during a break, I'm alone in the room and I pee, but what I actually leave behind is a pool of blood. You, the therapist, come in and gently reproach me while you mop the floor. But I'm mortified and don't say anything.

In therapy, Lisa says "It strikes me how much pain I felt," and the rest of the group observes that the dream occurs in the group therapy room, but she made everyone leave and was alone with the therapist.

In the clinical case described earlier, the group-environment is a space for the projection of shame. In the beginning, Lisa cannot speak while in group, she gets flushed and is subject to anxiety attacks if she is asked to speak. At the same time, the group is the first social environment in which she learns how to reveal her desires, loves, concerns, and attempts to get other women to like her as a woman. Once Lisa became comfortable with the group, she also began facing outside relationships with more self-confidence, and successfully reached the end of the therapeutic process, managing to separate constructively from the group.

Deconfusion techniques

Therefore, for the therapist, the strategic choice during the deconfusion stage is to assist clients in developing an awareness of their own transference processes. However, in order to do so, it is not enough to analyze what happens and what the client feels while in group. Indeed, it is crucial that the group as a whole become an oneiric matrix, in the words of Foulkes (1990) and Lawrence (1998).

This matrix is "a psychic network of communication which is the joint property of the group and is not only interpersonal but transpersonal" (Foulkes, 1990, p. 182).

According to Lawrence (1998), the regressive climate generated by the group facilitates the emergence of the Child ego state and the experiences precociously fixed in the script protocol. In such a climate, clients let the most archaic emotions come to the surface, like fear, excitement, shame, envy, guilt, and the desire to be important and perhaps dominate others.

Generating such a facilitating climate is the therapist's job and when they succeed, enactments, games, and dreams – themes around which are focused Chapters 13 and 14 – are also analyzed, along with free associations, core and lateral transferences. Among the Bernian techniques, the most useful therapeutic operations in this context are the ones that evoke the Child ego state, meaning illustration and interpretation. Therefore, it was crucial to be able to say to Lisa, in relation to her dream:

> In the past, peeing your pants was a consequence of the epileptic seizures, and it scared your mother and made you ashamed. Then, the same happened with the blood of your menstrual cycle. Now, you have brought your pee and blood inside the group and you don't feel ashamed anymore: You're human, you're a woman.

On this point, Tangolo (2015) writes:

> Such in-depth work implies relearning the functioning of the Child ego state which is new as far as pleasure, most archaic needs, the relationship

with one's body, and activating new neural circuits that trace new path-ways, are concerned. This being the aim, psychodynamic TA groups are probably the most effective tool, as they give an opportunity to work on different levels and create the most appropriate context both for relearn-ing and for choosing imitative – and therefore archaic – functioning strategies.

(p. 85)

The body in group

The experience of the group is profoundly corporeal: it recalls the archaic mem-ory of people reunited around a fire, the kind of comfort and anxiety caused by being in this magical circle of proximity. Groups physically reunite around a therapist in a room in which members breath, look at each other, and talk in a setting of intimate proximity. People can sit on armchairs or sofas, but are all close to each other.

On its own, such an intimate setting might lead to very different physical and emotional reactions between members. Some may start sweating, others blushing, and others might relax and feel safe.

The feelings of anxiety or safety caused by being in group, as well as the shame or pleasure of putting oneself at the center of everyone's attention are objects of analysis specifically at this stage of the therapeutic process, when the alliance is more stable and it is possible to deal with the most embarrassing topics.

Giulio's body in group

Giulio is 32 years old and is in therapy because he suffers from general-ized anxiety disorder and social phobia. He cannot have romantic rela-tionships and engages exclusively in paid sexual intercourse. He is rather ashamed of this and to the therapist inviting him to join a group he responds that he is afraid to become a monster and a serial killer of women and chil-dren. He does not know if he will be able to tell the group about these fears and troubles. After a few months, a fellow member plucks up the courage to tell him that his shoes stink and by being close to him she can smell them, and that makes her want to put some physical distance between them. Another girl says she has the same reaction and adds that when he talks about the trouble, he has to go out with women, her first thought is: "Of course, with that smell."

Someone worries that Giulio might be feeling terribly ashamed, but, to everyone's surprise, he cries out: "Ha! I finally got it. If *that*'s the problem, I could learn how to not be rejected."

Later, Giulio tells the group that he was rather neglected as a child, because his mother was depressed and often dirty, so she failed to take care of him or the house. It was very hard for him to learn how to wash and dress properly. Accepting the group's help and the feedback on his personal grooming, Giulio kept working on his pain and the feeling of inadequacy he had learned as a boy, due to which he felt "ugly, dirty, and bad."

On this matter, William Cornell argues (2015):

I have come to understand "armoring" as the interruption of the "spontaneous gestures" of both the somatic and interpersonal activities of the developing child – a child intent on both attachment and differentiation.

The transferential worlds that patients so often bring into psychoanalysis and psychotherapy are those of thwarted gestures interrupted by indifference, neglect, punishment, shame, violence, trauma, and failures within our foundational love relationships.

(pp. 96–97)

References

Berne, E. (1961). *Transactional analysis in psychotherapy: A systematic individual and social psychiatry*. New York: Grove Press.

Berne, E. (1966). *Principles of group treatment*. Oxford: Oxford University Press.

Blackstone, P. (1993). The dynamic child: Integration of second-order structure, object relations, and self psychology. *Transactional Analysis Journal, 23*(4), 216–234. doi:10.1177/036215379302300406

Cornell, W. F. (2015). *Somatic experience in psychoanalysis and psychotherapy: In the expressive language of the living*. Hove, East Sussex and New York: Routledge.

Foulkes, S. H. (1990). *Selected papers: Psychoanalysis and group analysis* (1st ed.). London: Routledge. doi:10.4324/9780429479847

Lawrence, W. G. (Ed.). (1998). *Social dreaming @ work*. London: Karnac Books.

Little, R. (2006). Ego state relational units and resistance to change. *Transactional Analysis Journal, 36*(1), 7–19. doi:10.1177/036215370603600103

Luborsky, L., & Crits-Christoph, P. (1990). *Understanding transference: The core conflictual relationship theme method*. New York: Basic Books.

Moiso, C. (1998). Il setting in psicoterapia di gruppo. In M. Novellino (Ed.), *L'approccio clinico dell'analisi transazionale*. Milano: Franco Angeli.

Tangolo, A. E. (2015). *Psychodynamic psychotherapy with transactional analysis: Theory and narration of a living experience* (A. Iozzelli & K. Jones, Trans.). London: Karnac (Originally published in 2010).

10

BASIC TECHNIQUES

Therapeutic operations

"Frustra fit per plura quod potest fieri per pauciora."
(Ockham's razor)

In *Principles of Group Treatment*, Berne describes the intervention a therapist makes in conducting group sessions or interviews which aim at the change they wish to achieve. "Taking as the most general statement that psychiatric patients are confused, the goal of psychotherapy then becomes to resolve that confusion in a well-planned way by a series of analytic and synthetic operations" (Berne, 1966, p. 213). In this chapter, Berne briefly describes, with brilliant logic, how a transactional analyst conducts the dialogue in order to attain decontamination and deconfusion. Therapeutic operations are thus specific transactional stimuli that the therapist proposes to the client in order to get rid of their confusion and to be oriented in the world of their own impulses, chaos of emotions, and primordial passions; in short to go from chaos to cosmos. Berne does not describe, in this context, the preliminaries of the interview or the group which comprise the transactions of encouraging, invitation to speak, and creating the atmosphere, which he describes in the first chapters of the book (e.g., "Well, tell me what makes you think so," or "Tell me what made you decide to come here, tell me something about you").

Therapeutic operations are all the interventions and interpositions aiming at bringing about change during the interview or the group session. The intervention is an operation on material brought by the client, while with the interposition the counsellor or the therapist adds new material. Let's imagine meeting a client who admits she has a problem of compulsive shopping. Let's try to examine how an effective interview might be conducted with this client according to Berne's operations. Of course, the interventions described in the following are not intended to be a sequence of interventions in the same interview. On the contrary, some of these interventions cannot and must not be precocious. It is necessary to understand and respect the level of awareness of the client, and the ego state activated in that moment, in order to decide whether one can proceed with interventions.

DOI: 10.4324/9781003215547-11

Interrogation

This is a question designed to receive an answer that, besides informing the therapist, invites the client's Adult to think and share material in the interview or in the group and that will later be used to work on the problem he has brought (e.g., "Do you know how much you spent on your clothes over the last month?"). The objective of interrogation is thus to make the contents explicit and straightforward.

> *Do* use interrogation when confident that the patient's Adult will respond.
> *Do not* use simple interrogation if it is likely that the patient's parent or Child will respond.
>
> (Berne, 1966, p. 234)

The problem with asking a client questions is that you cannot be too detached and inquiring. If the frequency of questions and the pace of the interview are emotionally in tune with the client, the therapist can enquire and hence know when it is time to ask and when to listen in silence.

Specification

This is a declaration on the part of the counsellor or the therapist, categorizing certain information. It may be confirming, as in non-directive Rogerian therapy (e.g., "So, you have always wanted to buy expensive things") or informative (e.g., "That's more of the little girl in you"). The objective of specification is to fix in the client's and the counsellor's mind certain information so that it can be referred to later without denials. Specification thus enhances awareness in the client, making him more aware about what he is communicating to us and sometimes causes insights (discoveries and intuitive illuminations) precious for the client.

> *Do* use specifications when it is anticipated that the patient might later deny that he said or meant something.
> *Do not* use specification if it will frighten the client's Child.
>
> (Berne, 1966, p. 234)

Increasing client awareness is the primary objective of specification. This operation enhances thinking and sharing the thinking co-constructed between therapist and client.

Using specification during an interview is like identifying some relevant points on the map in order to find our way through a confused bundle of information. Having the client involved in the reflection, which is possible thanks to simple and common language – like that used to describe ego states or to analyze transactions and games – is helpful in psychotherapy. It activates the client's Adult and helps to lay foundations for that essential co-operation in therapy which we define as therapeutic alliance.

Confrontation

This is an intervention on the part of the counsellor or therapist who uses information previously received from the client to underline inconsistency emerging during the conversation. This might disconcert the client's Parent, Child, or contaminated Adult, and put the client in a difficult position if the intervention happens at the wrong moment. It is an Adult – Adult transaction (e.g., "You are telling me that the situation is under control, but earlier you said that you don't know how much money you have in your account. How can these two things coexist?").

The objective of confrontation is to energize the uncontaminated part of the client's Adult. A thoughtful silence, or laughter due to an insight, indicate that such an objective has been attained. It is, however, a manifestation of the activation of the Adult, finally free from contamination.

> *Do* use confrontation if the patient is . . . playing "Stupid" . . . or if you are genuinely convinced that he is incapable of tagging the inconsistency himself.
> *Do not* use confrontation when it makes you feel smarter than the patient.
>
> (Berne, 1966, p. 236)

Confrontation is a key passage of the therapeutic session. It is not at all easy to set up confrontation on an Adult–Adult level: it is much easier to enter a judgmental dimension about inconsistencies in what the client is saying/the client's speech. What enables a therapist to set up confrontation at the right moment and use it as an opportunity for the client – rather than as an operation of "unmasking the guilty" or scolding the client as a parent – is a true non-judgmental attitude in the therapist's mind. If the therapist is sincerely interested in understanding and analyzing the strange and apparently incomprehensible balance among thousands of contradictions, this constructive process can begin. From my direct experience, it is mostly the intuitive activation of the Little Professor (archaic nucleus of Adult ego state or Adult in the Child, called A_1) in the therapist which enables the Adult meant as A_2 (second-level Adult, who can have second-order logical thought) to establish confrontation conducive to thinking, smiling, and perhaps even insight in the client.

Explanation

This is an intervention on the part of the therapist or counsellor that strengthens, energizes, decontaminates, and reorients the client's Adult—for example

> At the moment, you are playing "Yes, but . . .", so perhaps you don't really want the advice you are asking me for. A part of you does want to concentrate on therapy, but another one encounters many obstacles to setting up the next meeting.

or

> You have told me that after three months in which you had no money left in your account, you stopped going out and even paying for therapy and medicines to punish yourself. Can you see that when the Child takes over and becomes hyperactive, your Adult disappears and your internal Parent punishes you by deciding not to buy even something helpful for your health?

The objective of explanation is to provide the Adult, free of contamination, with precious information and nourish it in order for the alliance to be strengthened. Berne says:

> *Do* use explanation at every opportunity when the patient has been properly prepared and his Adult is listening.
> *Do not* use explanation if the patient is still "Butting" (Yes, but, . . .), "Cornering" . . . or "Trapping."
>
> (Berne, 1966, p. 237)

Therapists are often inclined to give long explanations, sometimes expressed in a language that is not comprehensible to clients. If one decides, especially after a successful confrontation, that giving an explanation is useful, the explanation must be brief in order for it to be effective. A therapist who speaks too much makes the client passive, and this may give rise to games, as Berne clearly stated. Explaining what is happening is again an invitation to think, to give a name to experiences that are anguishing or hard to understand; it also helps to analyze experiences one has lived through, to start hoping that the most disturbing feelings and thoughts can at least be contained, and eventually to start hoping to change.

Illustration

This consists of an anecdote or an exemplification the counsellor or the therapist provides after a completely successful confrontation for the purpose of reinforcing the confrontation and softening its possible undesirable effects. It is an interposition, an attempt to interpose something between the client's Adult and their other ego states in order to stabilize their Adult and make it more difficult for them to slide into Parent or Child activity (e.g., "It's as if inside you there were a parent that locks the naughty child in their room, and the child jumps out of the window, stealing their parents' money and feeling very satisfied because they've tricked them").

The objective of illustration is to reinforce decontamination and obtain alliance with the Child, who receives permission to be freed from Parental restrictions and be creative.

> *Do* use illustration when you are sure that the patient's Adult is listening, that his expressive Child will hear you, that his Parent will not take over.

Do not use illustration if you are talking to a self-righteous or literal Parent (as with many paranoids). . . . Do not use it to elevate your own self-esteem by showing how clever or poetic you are. Do not use it in an attempt to rectify an unsuccessful confrontation.

(Berne, 1966, pp. 239–240)

Metaphorical language is evocative, it activates the Child ego state, prevents Parental judgment, and enables the therapist to deal with very delicate material with the due protections.

In his lesson about lightness, Calvino (1988) wrote that it is like approaching the monstrous Medusa walking backward and holding a mirror that reflects the monster, just as Perseus did, so as not to be petrified. I find it very helpful to use archetypical images in therapy, for example, from Greek mythology, as they belong to the collective unconscious of western civilization. Indeed, in every people, mythology expresses, through effective images and stories, the great archetypical conflictual issues. If people from different countries came to see us as therapists, we should study, just like an anthropologist, the myths and stories of the civilization they belong to in order to help them solve their individual conflicts. These archetypical references sometimes emerge spontaneously, as they are part of the client's consciousness, and it can be defined through the language of a work of literature, a film, or a song. Heroes and myths with whom we identify are always explored in the script anamnesis and are very effective images in approaching the client's inner world, just like dreams and reveries.

Confirmation

This is the operation through which the counsellor or therapist reinforces the Adult functioning by revealing new material brought by the client after confrontation and illustration. It, too, is an interposition, an attempt to strengthen the ego state boundaries (e.g., "Even with me, in therapy, your Child pressed you not to respect our economic contract, and in the first sessions you have often forgotten the money to pay me"). The objective of confirmation is to consolidate the decontamination process by adding new material that logically demonstrates what we have already stated after the confrontation. The client's Child can deceive even the most prepared counsellor or therapist. Confirmation can thus be an interposition that reinforces the confrontation of incongruences and contributes toward unmasking the Child. Quoting from Berne:

Do use confirmation if the patient's Adult is established strongly enough to prevent the Parent from using it against the Child, and the Child from using it against the counselor/therapist.

Do not use confirmation if the original confrontation was unsuccessful, or if the patient is "Butting", "Cornering" or "Trapping."

(Berne, 1966, p. 241)

Confirmation accordingly consists in using experiences we have shared, often in the therapeutic setting, in order to enable the client to connect and assemble what has been observed within the microcosm of therapy with what happens outside of it. According to such a view, the group setting is the most suitable setting to provide material for either confirmation or denial of hypotheses which have previously been formulated. The group gives us a chance to observe and analyze several social behaviors and interactions which we otherwise might only have imagined through the script distortion. Some clients accept confirmations and confrontations mainly from the others in the group, and mainly if they have a very conflictual and ambiguous transference toward the therapist and learn more easily in the group than in the individual setting. At this point, the client is decontaminated, and the therapist can proceed and crystallize the situation. If the therapeutic contract allows the therapist to renegotiate with the client how and whether to proceed, they can discuss with the client whether to crystallize and conclude this path with the relief of symptoms and an improvement of relationships or to proceed to help the client overcome confusion through psychodynamic interpretation.

Interpretation

This is an operation typical of psychotherapy, not to be carried out in counseling. Its purpose is to deconfuse the Child. In a therapy contract, the therapist can propose such an interpretation:

> When you behave like that, being so naughty, and let your angry parent punish you, you end up looking for a "fairy godmother" who magically rescues you and takes care of your bills and debts. In your fantasy this is maybe what you expect from your spouse and from me as a therapist, that we pay for you and unconditionally accept you.

The purpose of interpretation is to proceed to an analysis of the script, and this happens through the decoding of the cryptic material brought by the pathological Child with their regressive needs and tyrannical demands. Quoting from Berne again:

> *Do* use interpretation where and when the patient's Adult is on your side, when you are not directly opposing the Parent, and when you are not asking too much sacrifice from the Child or arousing too much fear of Parental retaliation or desertion.
>
> *Do not* use interpretation when the patient's Adult is not in the executive position or is not properly prepared or is not on your side; nor when it is your Parent or Child talking instead of your own Adult.
>
> (Berne, 1966, p. 245)

Interpretation is the central part of the analytic intervention. In psychodynamic therapy, it also comprises the analysis of the oneiric material and parapraxis, acting-ins (acted in the setting), and acting-outs (acted outside the setting). Again, it is up to the therapist to use their experience and knowledge to know when they can proceed with a client on an interpretative level, when the Adult is allied, the Parent is not judgmental, and the Child is not too scared. Personally, I consider it difficult to interpret unless the internal Parent is at least partially restructured and the client has partially interiorized the new Parent learned during therapy.

Crystallization

This is a statement from the therapist or counsellor to the client's Adult when they are in a condition conducive to change (e.g., "So now you are in a position to stop playing 'Cops and Robbers' or 'Let's pull a fast one on Joey' and manage your salary yourself if you want to"). In an existential sense, the therapist brings the client to a position to choose, to exercise an Adult option on his life, and, if some contents have emerged which require deconfusion, to choose whether or not to do it in order to overcome an impasse. Again, according to Berne:

> *Do* use crystallization as soon as you are sure that not only the Adult, but also the Child and the Parent of the patient is properly prepared.
> *Do not* use crystallization if the patient is showing renewed signs of somatic disease, or a sudden access of courage or depression leading him into obviously hazardous situations.
>
> (Berne, 1966, p. 247)

Other interventions: Made by the counsellor's or therapist's Parent

For Berne, transactional analysis requires the eight operations described earlier. He adds that in some cases it can be useful or even necessary to use different approaches, particularly with psychotic clients, with whom it is preferable that the therapist be a Parent rather than an Adult for quite long periods during the intervention.

Support: This basically consists in stroking. Its content is not relevant, what counts is that the client feels they are being encouraged. However, it is advisable that the supporting messages are protective and permissive (e.g., "Come on, you can make it").

Reassurance: In this case, too, the tone of voice and the attitude are more important than the content, and it works mostly if the client's Child feels unprotected (e.g., "It's good for you to do so").

Persuasion: This contains seductive elements (e.g., "Why don't you do it?"), and the therapist must be aware that they will have to face the consequences of the attempts to arouse in the other person a decision to seek a cure for himself.

Exhortation: For example, "You have to do it for your health."

Berne adds that there are techniques that are directed to the Child ego state, but also that one must be prepared if one wants to use them. He also adds that there is a "bull's eye" transaction in which there is a therapeutic effect on all the three ego states of the client; he says that this is ideal to be striven for.

The bull's eye transaction

The bull's eye transaction is a stimulus from the therapist that has an effect on the three ego states of the client simultaneously. It is very effective, and it usually starts the moments of deeper change when a redecision and a permission are being prepared.

> I understand how difficult it is for you to give up your usual certainties [establishing bond with the P], but you can safely try new paths [permission to the C] because today you are able to choose and protect yourself [recognition of mature A].

This message was proposed to Sara several times at the last phase of her psychotherapy.

References

Berne, E. (1966). *Principles of group treatment*. New York: Grove Press.

Calvino, I. (1988). *Six memos for the next millennium*. Cambridge, MA: Harvard University Press.

11

ADVANCED TECHNIQUES

The therapeutic operations described by Berne in "*Principles of Group Treatment*" form the basis of TA therapists' interventions. However, the complexities of group processes require a specific set of techniques and competences – until now only briefly outlined in the literature – which deserve, in our opinion, a few observations.

The social structuring of time

Berne built a model to describe the different forms by which people structure time in social settings (Berne, 1966, pp. 229–232).

Withdrawal, rituals, pastimes, activities, psychological games, and intimacy are the six options people have for structuring their time during social interactions. Following this observational model, the therapist can lead the group toward activities and intimacy after having given space to its spontaneous ability to self-manage through the different stages of social interactions.

In the beginning, members may be closed off in their own internal dialogue, keeping to themselves, as if they were in a lift or on the underground, physically close but separated from strangers to protect themselves, avoiding conversation and physical contact with those they might regard with disinterest or fear.

Some members may keep isolating themselves even after the conversation has formally started, or they might go back to it during a stressful moment, such as a silent pause, a very aggressive interaction, or when somebody is complaining.

Directing

As a matter of fact, the most difficult thing for a group therapist is not figuring out what to say or do, but choosing which directing-style to adopt in order to handle the ever-mysterious, tangled web of relationships. This implies letting transactions happen, using them in order to make clients aware of their social scripts in order for them to change their transactions so as to change their internal representation of themselves and others. To this end, it is important for therapists

DOI: 10.4324/9781003215547-12

to observe closely the group's initial pastimes and avoid joining in as much as possible. As in a Lewin's old T-group, in this first stage, the therapist remains almost passive while members deal with the anxiety of close contact by resorting to defensive ways of passing the time while trying to find out if they run the risk of getting hurt in this new transactional context.

Berne devoted a fascinating chapter of "*Principles*" (1966) to the first three minutes of group therapy session, inviting therapists to focus on the present moment, observe, listen, and get into the right mindset for group therapy: to compose themselves "for a unique experience, for nothing just like the impending meeting has ever happened before, and nothing just like it can ever occur again" (Berne, 1966, p. 74).

When group members enter the therapy room, they go from the waiting room's silence and isolation to the social rituals of greetings. A therapist who goes in a few minutes after the clients, will find that, in time, each group, will set up its own specific ritual greetings. As long-time members have already formed the basis of a group culture, they are the ones to establish them in the first place. For example, in some groups, everyone waits outside the room, some having a smoke and a chat until it is time to go in. In others, everyone enters right away and takes their position on the sofas always following the same specific rules, leaving each member their usual seat as if to avoid crossing an invisible line. In some groups, people only wave or nod at each other and then sit down in silence; in others, they kiss each other's cheeks or shake hands.

After ritual greetings, therapists officially start the session, and from that moment on, they compose themselves in attentive silence. This silence sparks members' anxiety, who then cope with it in different ways. Some remain silent and wary, waiting to be addressed, others ask permission to talk about themselves or they start talking right away. When the group has already a history of shared interactions, this first moment can be used to connect the present session with the previous one. This proves to the therapist that the group is able to activate members' scripts and that everything is going according to plan: now the therapy can really start. This is where technique – that is, what to say or do within the context of members' spontaneous interactions – really becomes important.

The main directing technique in group therapy is to let things run their course, acting every once in a while as Parent in group interactions. Therapists can thus take on at different times the roles of "mother" or "father" at the family table and, while maintaining an observing Adult perspective, they can address members from a sometimes feared, sometimes desired Parent ego state. In such cases, however, the therapist will account for moments of meta-communication in which to examine what happened, so as to foster growth and development in the members' Adult ego state. So, in the beginning, therapists only make an appearance in clients' scripts, while later they explain what happens through Adult–Adult transactions, also shifting into a role of restorative and positive structuring Parent when deemed necessary.

Berne wrote that during pastimes, people look unconsciously for partners to play their games with. For this reason, therapists have to pay special attention to what may look just like the opening conversations of the proper group work.

"You're so lucky, you always get away with it so easily" is what a member (Person A) says to another (Person B) in an act of provocation, while they both enter the therapy room before the therapist's arrival. Person B reacts to this message with irritation, taking offense.

"See, she's always so bitter with me, she doesn't care that I'm in pain, she doesn't take me seriously." (thinks Person B without saying anything).

Person A acknowledges that she felt envious of Person B, because they are better than her at handling social problems and tackling the job market, while she has lost her job because she is depressed and feels more and more in a slump.

The aforementioned analysis of that initial remark was made possible because another member (Person C) was also entering the room and over-heard it. So, when the therapist came in, Person C thought it might be useful for the group to reflect on this exchange.

For the entire group, themes such as comparison, competition, and envy are very important, and Person A's provocation represented a good chance for everyone to work on themselves.

Thus, every transaction within the group is valuable and nothing can be simply thrown away. However, it is necessary to choose what to focus on and make a list of priorities so as not to get carried away: analyzing everything would be neither possible nor worth it.

Choices and priorities

Looking at the incredible amount of stimuli offered by members, therapists have to choose and follow the red thread of associations that allows them to orient themselves, much like Ariadne in the Minotaur's labyrinth.

A therapist's concern must be trifocal: an eye on the group process as a whole, an eye on each member's process, and . . . a third eye on the contents were discussed. Focusing on the frame, that is, the group's collective process, allows therapists to assess if the group is evolving in a healthy, physiological way, or if some energy is being blocked.

Tuckman's (1965) and Tuckman and Jensen (1977) stages of group development, as integrated by Clarkson (1992), prove themselves to be very useful to follow the group's cycles of growth and impasse, which are often connected to therapists' leadership style.

Therapists who work well in a group setting know how to provide the appropriate stimuli in order to allow a group's physiology to develop naturally. If, for example, the therapist proves to be ipercontrolling or ipernurturing, the group remains stuck in one phase: it might remain in a symbiotic, childish state without ever going through the storming stage, which plays a fundamental role in each members' identity formation process, as well as in helping them learn how to engage with others through Adult–Adult interactions.

On the other hand, if the therapist leads with excessively low energy levels and proves themselves incapable of giving enough strokes and stimuli, the group doesn't get to experience the natural symbiosis provided by a secure attachment, and thus risks never truly coming together as such.

Here, lay the major critical points for inexperienced therapists: assessing how and how much to intervene, how much to nurture, weather and when to speak or stay respectfully silent, and how much to observe from the sidelines or actively engage in the conversation.

How do you develop an adequate measure of therapeutic presence? How do you teach someone to be a group therapist?

It is not an easy recipe. The safest way is to learn through practice that is constantly recorded and supervised by a senior therapist. After an initial specific training on groups, it is also necessary to experience group therapy as a client for a time long enough to go through the entirety of the personal and collective evolutionary process, which takes about three years of clinical work. From that moment on, it is possible to start working setting up a therapy group to be recorded and supervised step by step. A confident leadership style develops in time: in fact, it is usually after a long period of training – both theoretical and practical – and after having weathered the first "storm," that therapists feel ready to embrace the uncertainty of group processes as if ready to sail the open sea.

Embracing uncertainty

Much like steering a ship at sea, the group therapist suggests a course and guides the navigation, teaches how to stay on board and how to avoid seasickness, but they can't predict what will happen at the specific intersection of destinies and scripts they helped bring together. There are so many variables that, even after a good clients' selection and preparation, it would be impossible to predict with certainty what will be. Embracing uncertainty is what Bion (1970) described – borrowing from the poet John Keats – as negative capability: that is the ability to deal with one's own anxiety as well as other's.

Many therapists don't work with groups precisely because they are afraid of not being able to control what happens, thus missing the fascinating and healing experience group therapy has the potential to be. A long clinical experience offers therapists the reassurance that they need to navigate these unchartered waters, since they have already encountered many bizarre social situations, and have learnt to orient themselves to survive the intricacies of the group's interactions, transactions, and games.

At the beginning of the 1980s, when I was a young psychologist-in-training, I lived for a year in a therapeutic community for drug addicts.

The Italian national health service hadn't yet started treating drug addicts, and the whole effort was delegated to voluntary organizations, which imported from the United States the Synanon's and Daytop Village's models (Yablonsky, 1988).

The HIV infection had landed brutally, ending lives and spreading fears among young addicts. In this context, communities were safe spaces where they experimented with any kind of group therapy, but, more than anything else, there was also a strong affective cohesion and the willingness to support each other. The groups I led during that time were a fundamental training ground, in which I learnt how to listen and observe, how to lead with authority and resolution toward appropriate behaviors those who wanted to beat each other up or throw themselves out of windows. I will be forever grateful to the people who taught me how to stand by the anguish of those who fight every day to find meaning in their lives while battling emptiness and despair.

When I'm in a tough spot during a group session I'm reminded of Letitia, who started running after another member to beat him up and whom I had to physically stop, or Maria, who wanted to leave throwing herself out of a window of the fourth floor, and stopped only when I started yelling.

In these adventurous group sessions, I learnt how look inside me and find the reasons to go through my own therapeutic process, as well as to start the transactional analysis training that allowed me to build myself a compass to navigate successfully.

Leading the group toward maturity

Following Clarkson's (1992) model, therapists act as leaders, offering small stimuli from the very first session in an effort to build the group up. Indeed, it is during that session that they gather for the first time a group of strangers together in the same room (going from a minimum of four people to a maximum of 8–10).

The therapist's aim is to create an environment where clients can recover *through*, but also *within* the group. Thus, it is necessary to explain to them how social interactions work in that particular context, spelling out the rules of group setting, and inviting members to introduce themselves and be open to giving and receiving feedback. It is also necessary to explain the reason why there is a whiteboard in the room, asking people to recognize the basic language of transactional analysis: each member is expected to give space to all of their three ego states, in order to find a more constructive way of being with others and improve their own internal monologue.

People choose group therapy because they want to be welcomed and not judged, to be listened to, and empathized with, but it is also possible to find within the group itself the same judgements and conflicts that characterized the member's outside interactions.

Members are not required to be good and non-judgmental, or to absolve anyone from their "sins": they are required to listen, to put some effort into understanding other people's reasons, and to be honest in giving feedback, even if it does contain judgements at times.

It will be up to the therapist to encourage everyone to recognize their own prejudices, illusions and phobias, or, in technical terms, the contaminations of their Adult ego state.

If therapists have an attitude that is open and welcoming of diversity, the group will model itself after this openness, especially in the first stage, when members, seeking inclusion, will put more effort into social behaviors that are compliant with the authority.

So, if the therapist asks members to come clean and sober to group therapy, everyone will accept this "rule" without questioning it, and someone will take it upon themselves to confront and challenge those who break it. By the same logic, members will be compelled to show up and be on time, as well as to justify a possible delay, in case the therapist requires to do so.

When people feel welcome enough, the group will be able to start talking as a "we." At that point, everyone will have found a stable sense of cohesion. Only then will it be time to move on to the next stage.

"What is my place?" The second stage is the storming stage, useful to define each individual's space inside the group. Here, a well-prepared therapist succeeds in encouraging conflict expression, which in the beginning manifests itself in a subtle manner. For example, a member's conflict style might involve taking up the whole conversational space for themselves. This is a kind of competitive client who starts talking and seeks to hold everyone's entire attention for most of the time, exactly as if they were a greedy child stealing other people's cake. Faced with this aggressive behavior expressed through a torrent of words, someone responds requesting that the therapist set rules and divide up the speaking time: for example, Terry suggests assigning ten minutes each, so that everybody can have a chance to speak (her life's motto is *Together apart!*).

Another member tries instead to intervene commenting everything that is said and bringing it back to themselves: "I also have a similar experience" and "Actually, for me it's" This way, they systematically intend to lead everyone's attention back to themselves.

This period of time in which members are trying to define their space and role within the group is very valuable because it allows therapists to get to know aspects of their clients that they had never had a chance to observe in an individual setting.

As therapists, we can here experience the strategies the client's Child uses to receive strokes, to beat the competition in the race for parental attention, and, in general, all the techniques clients employ to affirm themselves and try out their own power. However, this all makes sense only if therapists expose the connections between these behaviors and the script apparatus and give meaning to the stress of conflict: this way, members will be more willing to engage and share less "pleasant" parts of themselves with others.

At this point, the group is ready to move on to the next stage, where, on the one hand, they pursue mediation, confrontation, and interdependency while, on the other, they enact the deepest script patterns.

During this time, members acquire the more complex ability of coping within the group, learn to express themselves, come in conflict with each other, and mediate as adults to find suitable rules for a peaceful coexistence. At the same time, while on the one hand, they double down on their tendency to act on their until-then-implicit conflicts; on the other, they also reinforce their seduction techniques.

It is as if members unintentionally activated their Adult ego state on a social level (we have learnt how to act here, what the therapist and the others like or don't like), while on an implicit level, they in fact reactivated their Child ego state, or, rather were reenacting their Parent–Child script patterns. So, therapists might feel a sense of disorientation when faced with behaviors that would be hard to explain in another context. Almost everyone seems collaborative, satisfied, affectionate toward one another, and very much attached to the group. Yet, the number of "transgressions" is on the rise: suddenly, some members create a clandestine WhatsApp chat group to communicate outside the therapy setting, or two of them start a sexual relationship. Here, the therapy work grows deeper and it becomes necessary to give meaning to crises and transgressions through a deconfusion process. For therapists, it is fundamental to consider behaviors, manipulations, and tricks in the context of script fears, fear of change, and fear of breaking the pact of loyalty to the old Parent.

After making sense of this period of games, the fourth stage, centered on activities, becomes truly productive. In this stage, members bring inside the group their dreams, fears, and new behaviors, which are now recognized as efforts to solve archaic conflicts. They are more open and work mostly by themselves, with less of a need for interactions and stimuli from the therapist.

It is interesting to see the themes of transference analysis come up on their own: therapist and members appear in other members' dreams and in their daily musings. "The other day, while I was dealing with my boss at work, I thought of you and it helped me remember what you said during group session," someone might say, for example.

If therapists see the energy flowing this freely, they can choose to intervene only when they deem it necessary to express their point of view and reinforce an insight or a new behavior. It is during these happy times in which intimacy is more easily attainable, that the need to complete the therapy process starts blooming. This fifth stage, according to Tuckman, represents the conclusion of a formative process and a grieving moment, and it is different for each individual member. Clients leave the group one at a time, while others have to process the conflicting feelings related to this separation: "I'm happy for you, I see you're happy you've reached your goal, but you're leaving right when you've become pleasant for us all." "Now that we're finally comfortable all together, you're leaving," are typical expressions heard when somebody is saying goodbye to the group.

Therapists have to pay special attention to this stage every time it reoccurs because a member has completed their therapy process, or terminates it abruptly and prematurely: for each and every one, this is a great opportunity for therapeutic work.

We are not responsible for how we came into this world, but, very often, we are responsible for how we decide to leave it. Saying goodbye is a blessing that comes with the end of every therapy process, and the energy that results from a good conclusion, one that is not hurried nor delayed because of fear, is beneficial to both those who leave and those who stay.

References

Berne, E. (1966). *Principles of group treatment*. New York: Grove Press.

Bion, W. R. (1970). *Attention and interpretation: A scientific approach to insight in psycho-analysis and groups*. New York: Basic Books.

Clarkson, P. (1992). *Transactional analysis psychotherapy: An integrated approach*. London: Routledge.

Tuckman, B. W. (1965). Developmental sequence in small groups. *Psychological Bulletin*, *63*(6), 384–399. doi:10.1037/h0022100

Tuckman, B. W., & Jensen, M. A. (1977). Stages of small-group development revisited. *Group & Organization Studies*, *2*(4), 419–427. doi:10.1177/105960117700200404

Yablonsky, L. (1988). *The therapeutic community: A successful approach for treating substance abusers*. New York: Gardner Press.

12

MONITORING GROUP EVOLUTION THROUGH GROUP IMAGO ANALYSIS

Attaining change thanks to the group

Recognizing the client's internal images of themselves allows the therapist to diagnose the group script and thus follow and monitor group consciousness and the evolutionary development of group members. The group imago is any mental picture of the self in group, and of the group with respect to the self.

The experience of group treatment offers a chance to relive the building of one's personal identity through mirroring in attachment relationships and in peer relationships.

In the time spent together in the group, thanks to the stimuli from the therapist and the setting, the group represents a chance to walk along an emotional and cognitive path that is unique and powerful:

To relive, in a brief period of time, the history of how one's script has been structured;
To observe how survival decisions have been taken;
To understand how decisions can be changed so as to have a wider range of options and therefore a chance to be well;
To give up unrealistic objectives that are unattainable;
To experience that in the world there is space for oneself and for the other person, for every human being;
To learn how to achieve pre-established goals, in a constructive way both for oneself and for others.

The group treatment basically considers that the therapist observes how each member introduces themselves to the "micro-world" that is the group, and helps the client develop a group imago, the mental image one has about oneself in the group and the group in relation to oneself.

In the concept of imago and its use in Berne's type of group lies the essential tool of a transactional analysis therapist.

Group imago is a concept illustrated by Berne when he describes the dynamics of groups and organizations as the mental picture of what the group is like that

DOI: 10.4324/9781003215547-13

every person creates for themselves when entering the group, and that contains fantasies and projections on to the group, the leader, and its members, projections due to past experiences, particularly to the primary group they belonged to (Berne, 1963).

That is to say, if I was welcomed when I was born because my parents had been waiting for me for a long time and really wanted to have me, and I was accepted into my parents' and my family's lives, I will probably expect from the new groups I will enter – at school, then at work or with friends – to be treated like that, and I will therefore be willing to enter new groups and perhaps be curious about new opportunities. The group imago might, in this case, contain the image of a warm, friendly place, where I have my own space, where I can find smiles, interesting stimuli, people who encourage and support me, as if I were already programmed to repeat experiences of exchange, conversation, and intimacy. A person with such characteristics is glad to enter a group, even a therapy group, although they probably do not really need to do it from a clinical point of view, since their experiences as a child have already created the emotional and cognitive condition and the behavioral maps for them to benefit as much as possible from being with other people. This person may ask to enter a group at a particular moment of their existence, perhaps to deal with a separation, process a mourning, or face a change. This is the kind of person we may meet on a training course, in counseling, or at the lessons of a master's degree, and the request that can be made to a psychotherapist is to be supported as a specific step in one's own growth. This person is very likely to be satisfied with psychotherapy, and our work as therapists with them will be completely successful, although we cannot really take credit for that. A person with a good coping strategy is able to learn from life and new experiences, if only they are stimulated. If a student loves learning, the teacher can even be just "OK." So, an "OK" honest therapist is good enough to cure a client who has inside them the capacity to cure themselves and to seize all the opportunities life offers them. On the other hand, it will take a really good teacher to motivate a student with difficulties. In this case, there must be a good teacher and a good therapist. Going back to the group and the concept of imago, the therapy group is like medicine or a treatment course for those clients who do not want to come to terms with difficulties or to enter the group.

A person who does not want to enter a group often has a negative group imago, and expects not be accepted or to have to fight for their space. They might be embarrassed, afraid they won't feel comfortable or understood, and might think "I am so different from the rest of the world that the group won't be good for me."

If I am a person whose birth was not so easy, for example, I was born as an unexpected child or after an unsuccessful abortion, or when my mother or some other member of my family was sick, I will probably intuitively feel that there is not enough room for me in the world. If, then, I am the third or fourth child, I may be afraid I will have to fight to have a seat, to speak or to be listened to, to be seen by my parents, and I may similarly perceive the group as too tiring. There are some people, however, who, being the first-born, have had to substitute their parents and take care of the youngest children. They may re-propose this script in their lives as group leaders in society, like a team leader at work; if asked to enter a group, they may say: "It's difficult for me to be in a group if I'm not the leader." So, people who have the illusion of also being the only child in the world, where there are actually several billions of us, cannot even conceive of the group, even as a place to recruit followers. A therapeutic goal will thus be that such a person agrees to enter a group and, most important of all, stays after the first narcissistic wounds or disappointments. To have a client imagine entering a therapy group is a very helpful exercise to enhance the diagnostic process. You learn a lot about a client when group therapy is proposed and when you have a chance to observe them interacting with others.

Help clients to enable their group imago to evolve

The therapist's task is to recognize and analyze the level of the imago of each member of the group, and, most important of all, to support each participant in having their personal imago evolve to more mature levels of development and interaction with others. The group is a perfect place for a work of deconfusion and redecision regarding deep script issues. This is also the most complex skill to acquire as a group therapist: to be able to use every event of the group as a tool to be linked with the individual contract and redecisional development that the person needs requires great competence and a lot of concentration. The question a therapist is constantly thinking of is: How can each group member use this stimulus?

Before beginning

A person is the first to arrive at the evening meeting, and there is no one else in the room yet. The therapeutic question is: How do you feel about this event, and how is this related to your personal history and your script? Even if an event is fortuitous and is not determined by your actions, the way you describe the event to yourself is indeed connected to your script, the way you interpret and decode the events.

The examples I am about to give correspond to the four basic existential positions that in TA are described as pre-logical, emotional positions that every person activates in every circumstance as a filter of interpretation of events, of their own and the other's position in the event itself.

We define the constructive position as the "I'm OK, you're OK" attitude, usually described by the + + scheme. This means having an assertive attitude in every situation and decoding ambiguous events as events to be understood, not necessarily threatening. We define the depressive position as the "I'm not OK, you're OK" attitude, usually described by the + + scheme. A person in a depressive position tends to feel responsible in every difficult situation with others, whom they tend to justify and absolve, while confirming the sense of guilt for themselves – and guilt will be the most recurring feeling.

We define the paranoid or projective position as the "I'm OK, you're not OK" attitude, usually described by the – + scheme. Those who are in a projective position always blame others and constantly defend themselves by being aggressive to the person who is talking to them, so as not to run the risk of being criticized or being seen making a mistake, which they cannot stand.

We define the futility position as the "I'm not OK, you're not OK" attitude, usually described by the – scheme. This is the desperate and passive position of someone who gives up any chance to improve their own life, has a negative vision of themselves and life, and does not trust anybody. Thus, in the scenario of setting a group meeting, a group member enters the room on time and finds no one there. What they will think, what emotions they will feel, and how they will behave, both in this circumstance and later, surely depends on the four different existential positions that act as a filter to interpret such ambiguous situations as the one described.

Some people might think:

"Well, I'm the first, I will choose the most comfortable place" (+, +), and others: "They changed the time and I have forgotten because I am a muddler, others can be organized, while I can't" (–, +), or: "Others are late, of course, and we will waste precious time for our work" (+, –), and some "What am I doing here? I should have stayed home. What a lot of time I'm wasting with people I don't care about and who can't help me!" (–, –).

Emotional reactions are thus connected to these different representations of the event: I feel at ease while waiting for the others (+, +), I become anxious and fret (–, +), or I start accumulating resentment, so I get angry (+, –) or I experience a sense of void and desperation (–, –).

What do you say after you say hello?

A person's behavior after the others arrive in the group, the way one says hello, and the first transactional interactions are thus activated in the ego state which will be mainly energized with the thoughts and emotions described earlier. The therapist will, therefore, already have a chance to observe interesting and significant differences between the participants in the first exchanges. The group begins when the people arrive, say hello, and sit down. The therapist usually arrives some minutes later, and the dynamic is activated when they take a seat: the group time begins from that very moment. As we saw in Chapter 7, Berne said that, at the initial phase, a group member perceives the group situation as an undifferentiated whole in which only one's own slot (narcissistic slot) and the therapist's slot (transference slot) are distinguished; the others are seen as a whole from which only later other figures will be differentiated as individual figures.

Indeed, at a phase of introduction into the group, one can observe that the new member addresses only the therapist, often looks in their direction only, and does not remember the names of other group members. The new participant usually asks the therapist about the rules to be followed, and expects to receive information and support from them. An evolution can be observed when the new participant will be addressed directly by a peer and when they begin asking for information, asking questions, and openly disagreeing on some points.

The passage to the conflict phase in fact indicates a positive evolution, as the person feels sure that they belong in that context and gives themselves permission to explore their own space, their power, as well as that of others. It is as if people begin to touch each other when they begin to confront each other; being willing to exchange, being awkward in doing it, or making attempts that are sometimes awkward and sometimes aggressive to search for a contact, are extremely important experiences. Until children push, bite, or insult each other, they cannot even learn what the limit is in interaction, and how convenient it is to negotiate. Negotiating, which creates conditions to get back to playing after a fight, is the most helpful art in life, an art that needs exercising in order to be refined. Preventing children from confronting each other means leaving them completely unprepared to face the conflict that they are inevitably going to experience in relationships. If it is true that adults must not overstimulate aggressiveness or be overprotective, then it is true for the group therapist as well. They will have to intervene so that the conflict will not degenerate and lead to offensive judgements and, at the same time, cannot stop any manifestation of conflicts – albeit sometimes a little inappropriate – because this might block the participants' learning. It is very helpful to analyze in the group how conflicts begin, and, especially when their beginning is not evident, it is important to invite the participants to make the latent conflict explicit and have the members experience that it is possible to negotiate and find a constructive use for anger on a social level.

A group therapist cannot be afraid of anger or prevent group members from expressing aggressiveness, either toward each other or toward their own person. If the therapist blocks this process, the group is stuck in a symbiotic dependence that is not conducive to evolution. For Berne, this is the second phase of group imago. When the group members elaborate the meaning of the conflicts, their imago becomes more and more differentiated, they have a chance to recognize others as peers, and live more experiences of exchange and projections through the exchange with them. A third phase is thus reached, in which interactions among participants increase, and psychological games among members are activated, as they proceed to a time structuring that is more and more determined by the search for strokes, deeper stimuli, and confirmation of the script. Those who enter this third phase prepare to reach deconfusion, if they are ready to accept confrontation about games and to energize the Adult in order to understand the meaning of feelings they have or roles they play in the group, just as they do in their external lives.

To the fourth phase, clients bring their dreams, in which the group and the therapist are present, the deepest script issues emerge, each member works on a very deep level individually, and emotional contacts and insights are frequent, even in the exchanges among participants. It is the phase of intimacy and activity. Gestalt exercises and the analysis of dreams are helpful because the person is bringing out the Child world in which they are immersed and into which they are willing to let archaic memories and primary decisions re-emerge.

The fifth phase is the phase of elaboration of detachment, which accompanies the path to awareness of introjection of the inner Parent as a good and protective parent. It is a phase in which telling about successes at work or in one's affective life external to the group helps as a confirmation of the change that has taken place and as an encouragement to leave the nest-group.

Living the Bionian aspect of the group:
The group as an organism

The path to awareness and elaboration of the imago is indeed an individual path in the group. Nonetheless, it is important for a transactional analyst to observe how the concept of imago can have a Bionian application, that is, it can also be used to describe certain phases of the collective process. A group based on Berne's theory is averagely semi-open, that is, it begins with a certain number of clients (from four to eight) and then, as someone leaves the group at the end of his path, new members enter. The time in which one is in the group is thus different, and the phases of personal imago can be differentiated. However, the group sometimes seems to function as a single organism, and the model of imago can describe the experience of collective projections. The therapist can, in fact, perceive that the group is not yet structured, or that it is entering the conflict phase, or doing pastimes, or finally producing a common result until it elaborates separation.

Tuckman and Jensen's model (1977), which – as we already saw – described group phases as collective phases starting from the analysis of training groups, can indeed be applied to the marathon groups – in which the number of participants is the same at the beginning and at the end – and only in part to the weekly analytical groups if we, as therapists, can keep in mind that two levels coexist: collective and individual. A mature group, for example, that is at Phase 4 on a collective level, and in which deep experiences and dreams are being analyzed, begins to indulge in the intimacy that has been acquired until one of the members announces that they want to end therapy. Someone in the group might be upset and confront the participant aggressively, telling them that they are not ready and their decision is premature. Accordingly, if the group seconds the person who is preparing to leave the group and suggests a correct perspective for the fear of the member who is afraid of separation, the group will proceed to Phase 5. On the other hand, if the group identifies with the fear expressed by the participant who is anguished by the ghost of separation, it might regress to the phase of games, Phase 3 or even Phase 2, the phase of conflict. It is very important for a group therapist to follow, on the one hand, the collective process influenced by the emerging of various levels of leadership and, on the other, the participants' personal situations. In fact, the latter never completely coincide with the collective process if the people are healthy enough and the group is not pathologically "psychoticizing."

The "psychoticizing" group is one in which everyone is convinced they feel the same emotions and live in a condition of collective fusion. This does not happen if the therapist is trained and the group is supervised, as it always ought to be.

A therapist cannot begin a therapy group unless during their training they have personally experienced the group as a client. Indeed, the intensity of the emotions to be dealt with, and the complexity of the data to be analyzed, could not even be perceived by someone who has not deeply experienced them personally.

In TA, the focus of group treatment is the development of the imago of the participants, which is required in order to achieve the contractual objective. The group analysis is helpful as a background and comparison between the individual's level and the level of the collective organism. Such a comparison is also a helpful element in making a diagnosis: for instance, a client who denies the perception of conflict when everyone else feels involved in it shows us how isolated that client is and how their defenses work, just as much as a client who remains alone in the conflict while everyone else has moved toward more intimate exchanges indicates that they are afraid of being close to others and establishing a bond with them.

Alessio's case

The only child from a working-class family, he begins therapy because he has been referred by the seventh psychiatrist who has followed him.

He is 28; he introduces himself by saying that his father died eight years ago, he lives with his mother, and works in the company where his father worked. He has been having treatment for depression since he was six; he has had periods of health alternating with long periods of distress, which have always been treated psychopharmacologically. When he began therapy, he was being treated with anxiolytics and antidepressants for depression with panic attacks. He had previously been diagnosed with childhood depression, then school phobia, and generalized anxiety disorder.

His resources:

1 Alessio has been working and studying since he was 20: he is a worker and works eight hours a day, then he studies at university.
2 He has chosen the civil service.
3 He has had three girlfriends and quite a satisfactory sex life.
4 He reads and he is politically active.

His difficulties:

1 He has not graduated yet, and he suffers a lot before exams.
2 He cannot have long-term relationships because he feels suffocated.
3 He is obsessed by the thought that his mother will die, makes her undergo medical check-ups, and does not want to leave his mother's house.
4 He is a lonely person, he gets bored, and he does not really have a social life.
5 He thinks that he will be unable to continue working and that he will end up alone in a psychiatric hospital.

I bring Alessio into the group after 15 individual sessions, in which he is mainly in his Adapted Child and complains. I find out, however, that although he introduces himself as a "psychiatric client," he hardly ever followed the therapies prescribed, and never told the doctors, although he was supposed to.

Alessio's first period in group

Provisional imago: He does not want to enter. He perceives and describes himself as different from everybody. In fact, he does not look anyone in the eye, he is on his own, he does not even listen, he is often distracted. When he asks to speak, he turns to me, the therapist, and says: "I want to tell you." He ignores the others and only looks at me.

Intervention: Unconditioned strokes, emphasizing adaptive behaviors, invitation to establish a playful contact with the others, confronting the incongruity (you come to the group, but you only speak to me: Shall I translate for the others?).

Alessio's second phase in group

Adapted imago: He is encouraged by the other members of the group to speak and exchange ideas with others; Giulia accuses him of being there without a role and of not being interested in others. Alessio is afraid of such direct stimuli, but he likes being addressed directly. He quarrels with some members of the group, jokes with others; the moments of contact with the members increase.

Intervention: Emphasis, specifications to stress the value of the energy of the Rebel Child, and the new experiences of exchange and contact.

Alessio's third phase in the group

Operative imago: A period of intense exchange begins. He asks me, as a therapist, "What do you think about me?", asking for confirmations, and playing "Wooden leg" and "Poor me" (Berne, 1964). After the summer break, he does not call me by name, he calls me "Doctor," as if he were seeing me for the first time. He is no longer on first name terms and asks for an individual session because he feels "terrible." In the confrontations in the group, he declares that he is angry because he felt that he has been "abandoned" during the summer, while he actually lives in his own house and he is doing pretty well. The comments from the group are affective and ironical: "Look, you're smarter than you think."

Intervention: Analysis of games and subsequently confrontations, emphasis, and specifications of new, realistic, adaptive behaviors, then illustration, confirmation, and crystallizations.

Alessio's fourth phase in the group

Secondarily adjusted imago: Period rich in experiences and intimacy in the group. Alessio feels part of the group, is nourished by the group's affection, he always sits close to someone, touches the others and lets them touch him. He speaks addressing every member, calls them by name, and tells them about his difficulties and achievements. He ends therapy after four years, having been free from medication and psychiatrists for three years; he has graduated, is autonomous from his mother, and has a steady love relationship and a group of friends.

Interventions: In some moments, each phase is reanalyzed in microsequences; interpretations and crystallizations enable Alessio to let the awareness and energy of the reparative here-and-now leave a sediment and stratify. The therapist is, for him, his mother; the group represents the world. The mother-therapist was for Alessio a dangerous and entangling place for relationships, in which he was drowned by evil fantasies and childish demands. Growing up implied loneliness and abandonment. In Alessio's experience as a child, there were no brothers or sisters or positive friends. The group becomes the world and a training place, a nurturing and nourishing place, but at the same time, a more realistic place to which to adapt himself. The group reactions represented the main factor for change for Alessio, providing him with new attachment patterns and opportunities. My initial intuition was: this child is too lonely, he cannot play with others, and he needs to learn to play, to touch, and be touched.

Terry's case

Terry is a woman aged 45; she is a clerk. When I met her, she has a husband and two children – Giulia, 13 years old, and Luca, nine years old. She began therapy when her daughter presented worrying adolescent symptoms of parental refusal, with violent threats to her brother and self-destructive behaviors.

Terry would say: "I'm here for my daughter," but then, every time she spoke, she spoke about herself. Her husband and her son were never part of her stories. She had a deep sense of guilt about Giulia: "I nearly killed her." When Giulia was four, her brother having been born a short time before, Terry was responsible for her daughter being in a coma due to a very high fever because she refused to take her to hospital, until her husband took the child from her. "Now she wants to kill me," she says in the first interview. The therapeutic approach of the team for three years was to follow Giulia with both a pharmacological treatment and psychotherapy, and to follow her parents in a support therapy whose purpose was to reinforce their parental competences. As Giulia's behaviors became less worrying, and her parents managed to deal with both of their children, we accepted Terry's request to begin individual psychotherapy with TA. Giulia attends high school, is politically active, and has a boyfriend. She has completed the pharmacological treatment and is still seeing a psychotherapist; she will stop when she is 17 and start again out of choice when she is 20. Luca finishes lower secondary school, starts high school, and little by little finds his own space in his family. The father is the one who makes decisions about the relationship with the children, and he has a constructive, important role in Giulia's therapy too. The children tend to rely on him more than on their mother because Terry is very little involved in the decisions that concern them. Terry comes from a middle-class family, and her mother categorically rejects the children, whom she has never hugged and with whom she shakes hands as if they were strangers (she seems to have a serious narcissistic disorder and to propose an avoidant attachment). Terry does not remember much about her father. Terry is apparently cold, with a gelid anger; only Giulia's emotional impetus seems to touch her. There is not enough room for everyone in her family of origin: her mother takes up all the space. At work and in her family, Terry feels as if she is not there: "I'm like a shadow. I don't decide anything. I don't say what I think, I don't say what I want." However, as her husband declared in the therapy for the parental couple: "We really are all subjugated to your will, we only do what you want us to do." Terry is introduced into a group after a period of individual treatment. We are currently at the final phase of her treatment, and the following reflections come from an exchange between Terry and me about her path in the group.

Terry's first phase in group

Provisional imago: She does not want to enter, she feels different from the others and defines herself as such. In fact, she does not look at anyone, she sits aside, she does not even listen, and she blushes if someone asks her something. When she asks to speak, she turns to me, her therapist, and says "I'm going to tell you." She ignores the others and only looks at me. She clearly shows that she is not listening to the others and that she gets annoyed if she cannot speak. She agrees to listen to the others – if they do not take too much time, and only provided that she has had a chance to speak herself. She would like to divide up the time by assigning just a few minutes to each of the others to speak.

Intervention: Unconditioned positive recognition, emphasis on adaptive behaviors, invitations to establish a playful contact with others, and then confrontation about incongruity (you come to the group but you only speak to me: Shall I translate for the others?).

Terry's experience:

> At the beginning I'm very curious, and I'm attracted by novelties. S. bothers me because she speaks too much, what she says is no use to me, she deprives me of my space. K. also bothers me, because she is not sincere and when she speaks she deprives me of my space. When I speak I like it, I calm down, I feel I'm really there, but at the same time I feel guilty because I'm depriving someone of their space. Meanwhile, immersed in this uneasiness, worried about not having enough space, I don't enjoy the novelty, I don't participate and unless I have previously spoken, I can't understand anything of what the others say.

Second phase

Adapted imago: She starts complaining because there is not enough space for everyone. She would like the time for speaking to be equally shared. She cries (out of anger, she will say) if there is no time for her. She wants to be seen by me, the therapist, and if she is not explicitly asked to speak, she threatens to quit. She fights with some in the group, jokes around with others, and the moments of contact increase.

Interventions: Emphasis, specifications to stress the value of the energy of the Rebel Child, and the new experiences of exchange and contact.

Terry's experience:

> It bothers me that each member of the group, including the thera-
> pist, always sits in the same seat. It particularly bothers me that
> K. got the armchair. I would like, once in a while, to sit in E.'s
> [therapist] armchair and the places to be rearranged. It bothers me
> that we start late because of E. [therapist], and I feel relieved when
> someone in the group is missing. The fewer, the better. Maybe this
> is what I want most, so it is more likely that there is space for me.

Significant changes:

> After never-ending doubts and second thoughts I decide to attend
> a residential training group in the summer, I take my own space.
> I join a drama group and I begin to express myself. I feel part of a
> small group of colleagues.

Third phase

Operative imago: A period of intense exchanges begins. She asks me, the
therapist, "What do you see in me?," she asks for confirmations, wants to
know how important she is for me. She expresses competitive behaviors,
the games she activates in the group are "Schlemiel" and "If it weren't
for you." She asks for individual interviews, then compares group therapy
with drama experiences and considers therapy a less valuable experience
if compared with drama, as in a competition (it is more helpful than you).
In confrontations in the group, her anger emerges because she does not
feel as if she is a protagonist and she does not feel she is being sufficiently
helped, although she actually receives a lot of strokes. The comments from
the group are affective and ironical: "Look, you're still with us!"

Interventions: Analysis of games and then confrontations, emphasis, and
specifications of new behaviors, realistic, adaptive, then illustration, confirmation, and crystallizations.

Terry's experience:

> Moving to a new study [the group moved to a larger study] meets
> my need to have an armchair of my own. I take it. I like sitting in
> the same seat, I like that place to be mine. I'm still critical about
> E. [therapist] I'm not sure she is the right person for me. I keep
> an emotional distance from her and I don't feel she is friendly to

me. I think what I'm doing with her is not enough, so I keep going to the training courses I started, and I take up a therapy based on spontaneous movement. It seems that these three things together are helping me. I would like, also in the group with E., to have experiences of exchange, in pairs, in threes, all together, I would like to create a relationship with the other members of the group. I'm critical about the "speak one at a time" policy, one can start only after the other has finished – this way there is no interaction. I would like to share what I've experienced outside the group, but I don't. I need someone to give me permission to do it, it would take time and I don't know if the others are interested. I just let E. get the message "You're not doing enough." I express the idea to quit therapy, and I'm glad that E. won't let me go. I begin feeling present and part of the group. I always need E. to give me permission to assert myself and to express what I'm feeling. At the same time, I feel more comfortable when there is only C. [co-therapist] to conduct the group. Meanwhile, thanks to my drama experience, I start being visible, and I occupy my own place on the sofa and in the group. I feel under the spotlight.

Significant changes:

I find myself the protagonist in a theatre production. I find myself facing the fact that not everyone likes me, and I accept that. I'm perfectly comfortable when the group becomes smaller, I feel surrounded by the intimacy that has been created. My daughter leaves our house and goes to live on her own. From inside me emerges the idea that there is something buried down deep and removed.

Fourth phase

Secondarily adjusted imago: A period rich in experiences and intimacy in the group. Terry feels part of the group, she is close to the others, looks at them, and lets others look at her. She speaks and addresses everyone, calls the others by name, and talks about her achievements and her difficulties. She often brings her dreams and her drawings, in which there is always the group and a wall falling down.

Interventions: At some moments, we analyze all the phases in micro-sequences, interpretation prevails, and ancient memories of childhood and ancient traumas re-emerge.

Terry's experience:

> I'm closer to my husband, and I wish to meet him. I'm not so
> uncomfortable about his anger, or the thought that he is going to
> get angry at me and doesn't understand me. I feel fine when he is
> here too. New people are introduced in the group, and this attracts
> me, rather than bother me. I can participate even if I never speak in
> a whole meeting. In the drama group, I always express my anger.
> I'm more and more aware that for me the relationship with others
> is a fight for power, "either you or me . . ." [she cries as she says
> this and marks the sheet with a tear]. Either I prevail, and judge the
> other, don't listen to them, or I abandon the field, and get revenge
> through emotional distance. There isn't space for me and the other
> together. I feel the need to inquire deeply into my relationship with
> my parents, with my husband and with E.

Significant changes: "I spend a week alone with my husband and I'm
perfectly at ease. We talk, and he says he feels fine too."

Currently: Fifth phase

Terry can prepare herself to leave the group, she must be free to take the
time she needs to separate. She is coming for some individual sessions to
re-elaborate her path, and then she talks about that in the group. Commenting on Terry's path, I reflect on the fact that I proposed that she enter the
group quite early because individual treatment was more difficult for her,
she had a negative transference full of cold anger toward the therapist and
she would probably have quit therapy. The mother-therapist was for Terry
an unknown and feared place for relationship, from which she escaped. One
of her first memories is dancing alone in the living room. She remembers
the rooms and the house but not her mother's presence. Her father, who
was more affective, has been suppressed from her memory. Growing up
meant freeing herself from an oppressive absence-presence (her mother was
a painter and filled their house with her paintings). In her childhood experiences, there weren't any positive friends, brothers, or sisters, although she
does have two brothers – but with them, she hardly had a relationship. As
it happened with Alessio, for Terry, too the group becomes a world-training
place, a nourishing and nurturing place, but at the same time a more realistic place to adapt to, a place to be feared because there is no friendly,
welcoming place to go back to. Terry had run away from her family when
she was 20, as soon as she had a chance. The group relationship offers her

new attachments and new opportunities, and they are the main factor for change for Terry.

My initial intuition had been: this woman will not be able to be a mother unless she is accepted as a child and her trauma is healed. "I am a bad mother who didn't want her children, who nearly killed them and would want to get rid of them now." In another episode, she remembers that she had to cross a road with her two children; each of them was on a different bicycle. She sent them forward and remained on the sidewalk, without protecting them, and then felt guilty at the thought that a car could hit them. Her mother is a bad mother too, she never hugs her children and always shakes hands with them as if they were some strangers she had just been introduced to. The therapist is perceived as bad, too, and Terry does not feel wanted: "Perhaps you're not the right person to take care of me," Terry would say to me. The sentence: "There isn't space enough for you and me" always resounds inside Terry, and it means: For me and my mother, for me and my daughter, for me and my husband, for me and my son, and for me and the group.

> Therapist, and what about you, have you got a place for me? The group can be a welcoming womb: You and I in the warmth of other people close to us, it can be the place where we see ourselves mirrored in others, where we learn to express our emotions and to be close to the parental figures.

It is to the group that Terry brings a lot of dreams, elaborates the deepest experiences, and then asks for individual sessions to reanalyze the emotional material that the group so richly aroused. The important dreams say that in this place, anguish ends and a bag is found that was always lost.

References

Berne, E. (1963). *The structure and dynamics of organizations and groups*. New York: Lippincott.

Berne, E. (1964). *Games people play: The psychology of human relationships*. New York: Grove Press.

Tuckman, B. W., & Jensen, M. A. C. (1977). Stages of small-group development revisited. *Group & Organization Studies*, 2(4), 419–427. doi:10.1177/105960117700200404

13

TRANSFERENCE, COUNTERTRANSFERENCE, GAMES, AND ENACTMENTS

In this chapter, we will analyze the topic of games in a group setting according to a transactional analysis approach. We will see how the theory of games was subject to several changes since Berne, how it could be likened to the concept of enactment, and, as a consequence, how the therapist's personality is involved into the transference–countertransference matrix relation. This theoretical model will be extended to the group setting, focusing on transference and countertransference dynamics and the implicit regulation of emotional experiences. The clinical cases presented in this chapter will provide examples of shared group regressions, which evoke script dynamics and allow the reorganization of the clients' intrapsychic structure through the discovery of new ways of being in group. The last section will focus on the therapist's countertransference responses and the group members' lateral transferences with respect to the individual client's level of psychological functioning and personality disorder.

Games and enactments

"Thanks for playing my game" is one of the final lines Mark Rylance's character says to the protagonist of Spielberg's *Ready Player One*. This line suggests a concept of game as understood by many authors operating in the field of TA.

According to relational psychotherapy, therapists are not merely neutral observers of the client's intra-psychic world and behavior, but, in line with Heisenberg's uncertainty principle of quantum mechanics, because of their role as observers, they are already necessarily interacting with – and thus influencing – the object of their observation. Therapists' participation and involvement are not considered obstacles to eliminate, but are seen as crucial elements of the therapeutic action. Without therapists' participation in clients' games, psychotherapy could become artificial and lack an authentic interplay, risking to trap both clients and therapists in predefined roles.

When therapists listen to clients, they are listening to a big part of themselves as well, and through their subjectivities they are able to contain and process what comes from clients: a therapeutic relationship involves two stories – both of which include scripts, affections, values, and thoughts – intersecting and

DOI: 10.4324/9781003215547-14

influencing each other, bestowing on the clinical process its mutable nature and form.

If therapists accept to influence clients and be influenced by them, enactments, meaning the therapist's participation in the transference, may constitute a door to otherwise impenetrable areas of the client's personality. It is about playing together, creating a space in which the intra-psychic may be connected with the interpersonal, "thus [therapist and client] can become aware of the repeated elements and understand the therapeutically needed relationship" (Little, 2006, p. 17). We use the term "enactment" and not "projective identification" because we want to take into account the relational setting in which the unconscious communication takes place. In fact, in this case, the therapist is not regarded as a container of the components projected onto them by the client, but they are an active participant, with their specific subjectivity, of the therapeutic process.

According to Novak (2015), games and enactments, despite several similarities, are to be considered as separated constructs. Games are a defense against unconscious experiences, while enactments reveal unsymbolized unconscious experiences.

Stuthridge (2015) argues, instead, that games and enactments are not exactly synonyms, but have several elements in common. According to her, enactments take place when a player excludes the complementary role and provokes it in the other, creating split complementarities such as accuser and accused, persecutor and victim, seducer and seduced, and betrayer and betrayed.

Enactments are described using Karpman's (1968) Drama Triangle in the PDM-2 (*Psychodynamic Diagnostic Manual*, Lingiardi & McWilliams, 2017), as well: as a result of a client's childhood trauma, in which there is a perpetrator and a victim, therapist and client may experience the same or opposite roles (the client may take on the role of the persecutor and the therapist that of the victim) in the course of the therapeutic process. Thus, the Drama Triangle offers a useful contribution in order to comprehend the transference–countertransference dynamics of trauma.

Berne (1964) defined games as "an ongoing series of ulterior transactions progressing to a well-defined, predictable outcome" (p. 48). According to Chang and James (1987), "a game is an attempt to deal with the intra-psychic conflict projecting it onto the outside, so as to relieve anxiety and control the conflict itself" (my translation, Novellino, 2004, p. 126). Games thus reveal communicative barriers, enacted unconsciously in a repetition of ancient modes of relation – learned during infancy in order to receive attentions and recognition – as if living in a sort of "remembered present" (Edelman, 1989).

Jacobs (1986) defined enactment as "transference enactment": the client tends to persuade the therapist to take part in unconscious and silent games which filter into the transference–countertransference matrix.

The descriptions of games and enactments reveal unconscious and intersubjective processes: as we have seen in Chapter 4, these processes involve two minds communicating unconsciously and synchronically right brain to right brain at a nonverbal level through emotional transactions (Schore, 2020).

According to Stuthridge (2015), Berne's ego states theory lends itself to an interpretation of the mind as a multiplicity of non-linear self-states which force us to face contradictory inner experiences that we are often unable to integrate. The Parent and Child ego states, again according to Stuthridge, are akin to actors in a play, who, with their behaviors, feelings, and thoughts, associate and interact freely and flexibly with each other, within both the inner world and the outside relationships of the whole person, following the Adult's guidance. The latter, like a stage director, arranges and coordinates in a harmonious way the different characters. However, in the case of developmental trauma, such actors remain more or less dissociated, each one acting unbeknownst to the other: the boundaries between ego states are rigid and hinder connection.

Games and enactments represent a dramatization of the dissociated ego states, a sort of live theatre in which it is necessary to recognize the meaning of the setting in order to be able to understand precocious traumatic experiences, "revealing unformulated experience that require us – in the midst of confusion, shame or guilt – to reflect on our own participation, often aloud with the patient" (Benjamin, 2017, p. 145).

Thus, through games and enactments between client and therapist we can observe a relationship in which the original trauma is reactivated, creating complementary dualities such as: "You or me," "Your way or my way," and "Who acts and who is acted out." The game of "Why Don't You – Yes But" is the perfect example, as it manifests a position in which, metaphorically, only one mind can survive the other. In it, each player firmly stands their ground, dissociating from the awareness of sharing some aspects with the other. By processing enactments, it is possible to move on, in the therapeutic relationship, from the game of "Why Don't You – Yes But" to the third position of "Yes, and . . ." or "Both . . . and. . . ." This is the moment in which the ego states in each participant's mind change in synchronous response to the encounter with the ego states of the other.

Enactments in group

In a therapy group, each member plays a role and "invites" the others to play their game, maybe interpreting different roles and enacting past experiences which have never been processed or understood up until that moment. Therapists, too, join the clients' games, letting themselves be involved into a whirlwind of unpleasant, intense, and vibrant emotions, pushing to access an intersubjective space. In such moments, the group process may appear fragmented and the transferences between members difficult to understand. In particular, when a client threatens to self-harm or carry out dangerous acts, therapists start to feel excessively responsible, not only with respect to the client in question but also for the entire group.

It is only when the therapist is able to make sense of what is happening that the group becomes a solid container capable of making all members, including the client who initiated the game, feel like coherent and defined subjects, because someone finally listened to them without being scared or shocked, and was brave enough to play their game with them. "Thanks for playing my game" is what each member might say after having experienced and processed enactments in group.

Clients suffering from personality disorders, who often carry a traumatic past on their shoulders, are particularly scared of the intimacy that might form within a group, and for this reason they tend to play the roles of monopolizers, scapegoats, or persecutors. When a traumatic experience is not inscribed in memory, the contents of that experience, which we might consider as nonverbal sub-symbolic elements (Bucci, 1997), are acted out by the client in order to find in the here-and-now that lost sense of self.

Enactments represent a challenge for both the therapist and members' reflective thinking skills. They are unexpected moments of particular intensity, in which members share stressful recollections characterized by rupture, repair, and interactive regulation of their dysregulated affections. The right brain's intense emotional changes experienced by one member might resonate synchronically in all other members and allow the therapist to encourage a group regression, moving from the conscious and known left brain to the unconscious depths of the right brain. "Recall, reenactments of attachment dynamics occur as transient clinical regressions into an earlier stage of development. Neuropsychologically, the group synchronously shifts dominance from later-developing left hemispheric verbal reason to early-developing right hemispheric nonverbal emotion" (Schore, 2020, p. 14).

Eleonora, a client suffering from dependent personality disorder, has been a part of the group for two years and has developed a good relationship with fellow members, four women to whom she has learned to open up about the many abuses she has suffered in her childhood at the hands of a neighbor who used to take care of her when her parents were not at home. Men are pretty much non-existent in her life. She has been living on her own for years and she manages to feel fulfilled only with regard to her career. When Andrea, a new member, joins the group, Eleonora reveals to him, too, the traumatic experiences of her childhood and describes the shame she feels around her body, as well as the subsequent terror at the idea of being touched by men. While she is still talking, Andrea cuts her off, vaguely irritated, and reproaches her for complaining, while at the same time urging her to take a look at herself from an outside perspective: she seems like a nice, open, and good-looking woman. He berates her for her feelings of inadequacy, and for letting a far-off past dictate limits to her present, irrevocably taking away her future. Andrea's wife often complains, as did his mother, who was abused and cheated on by her husband and suffered through all of it in silence without ever fighting back. Because of this, Andrea has always had a powerful "Be Strong" driver and thus tends to project on the outside his weakest, most fragile parts, which he dissociated from himself in order to survive a family context fraught with conflict. After these unexpected remarks, nobody, including the therapist, says a word. Everyone is confused and surprised, as if Andrea had uttered real words of affection and admiration toward Eleonora, but, at the same time, had dared to invalidate the pain she felt from her wounds. Eleonora is left speechless as well, her body completely still, an expression of pain and anger on her face. At times, her eyes dart to the therapist, who, after a few minutes of silence, flushed and clearly embarrassed, asks her: "What is it, Eleonora?" The words are thrown around without much of a thought, mechanically, as a way to relieve the tension caused by Andrea's remarks. Acted out, thought-less words. "What is it?" answers Eleonora in what is almost a cry. "You didn't say anything! You're not protecting me! He attacked me and you didn't say a word. . . . That's what it is!" Silence falls once again over the room.

The therapist feels that something that should not have happened is happening: she has become Eleonora's enemy, her bad object, and for the first time after years of therapy, the client is angry with her. A sort of enactment is taking place, where the group's right brain is communicating with Eleonora's, and in that palpable silence, we can almost hear the voices of all members' C_0, waiting for the therapist to save the day with her answer.

In such situations, it is as if time expanded, minutes of silence become hours, and the therapist, too, feels swallowed up in Eleonora's traumatized world, paralyzed with terror at the idea she suddenly turned into Eleonora's mother, unable to protect her daughter from her neighbor's abuse. She realizes in that moment that she never allowed herself to act spontaneously toward Eleonora, as Andrea had done. During the entire time of the treatment, she had always kept her Nurturing Parent activated, trying to set herself apart from Eleonora's real mother, who was cold and unloving to her, and identifying in the complementary role of the daughter (Novellino, 2004). The therapist's fear of further hurting a person already devastated by childhood trauma prevented Eleonora from expressing, and thus integrating, her aggressive emotions, contributing to keep her in the role of the victim.

While therapist and members are still speechless, Eleonora, feeling like she has lost the unconditioned support and approval of the idealized therapist, attacks Andrea, accusing him of being insensitive and lacking any tact, but also of invalidating her pain while concentrating exclusively on his own needs. Eleonora claims her right to be seen as a victim of a series of terrible injustices, which damaged her dignity as a person and as a woman. It is incredible how, observing Eleonora's fury toward Andrea, we can catch a glimpse of that dignity and life force that had seemed all but lost forever.

Reclaiming her right to be seen as a victim, Eleonora stops being one, because her vulnerability turns to strength.

The dissociated elements, the ego states relational units, are being enacted in a shared game: her Persecutor Parent, which until that moment Eleonora had turned against herself by overeating and neglecting her femininity, is now turning its perspective to the outside. Andrea refuses to retract his words and that makes her even angrier, as if each of them was trying to resist the other's claim.

When Sara, who is usually quiet and shy, confesses that Andrea gave voice to something she would have never dreamed of saying out loud for fear of hurting Eleonora's feelings, the tension within the group eases a little. Everyone collectively breaths out a sigh of relief.

The therapist, who had been paralyzed by guilt up until that moment, had shared the group's tension. However, after having analyzed what was happening and soothed her anxiety, she takes the floor and openly admits that she had always preferred to feel like a good mother toward Eleonora – thus avoiding having to recognize her true needs, which went beyond simply being rescued from her past – and had always tried not to be regarded as an enemy by the client. Andrea, a new voice in the group, allowed Eleonora's resourcefulness to emerge.

It is as if everyone in that room was fighting external enemies without caring about Eleonora and her ability to her anger to transform her relationship with men. Other members share Sara's and the therapist's opinions and the unsaid comes to the surface, the kind of unsaid that invalidated Eleonora's subjectivity and prevented the development of a shared reflection based on pursuit, discovery and integrating abilities.

Eleonora seems to sit up straighter on her chair while she listens to the therapist and the others talk, she is confused and surprised, but her expression is more relaxed and there is a new vibrancy to it. She listens to the others' words, especially those from the women she trusts, and looks like a little girl observing her friends play a game of which she does not yet know the meaning, but realizing there is more than meets the eye. This "more" might not be so dangerous after all.

During the following sessions it was important to draw Eleonora's attention on her stubborn and unwavering refusal to accept that Andrea also offered words of support and positive reinforcement, pointing out how her attention was entirely focused on what she had interpreted as a refusal to empathize with her terrible pain and suffering.

In the here-and-now microcosm, Eleonora started to become aware of how she had built her whole identity on that pain, distorting her perception of others, and especially men: The latter were all, in her eyes, insensitive and authoritarian – Andrea was the only man in the group – and this perception of them was the main reason behind her unwillingness to pursue romantic relationships with them. Women, on the other hand, were seen as loving and understanding, but only when they recognized her suffering. Pain had become a sort of contaminating agent which had intoxicated her body and soul, depriving her of all hope of change, as well as of her capacity to take responsibility for her own life.

Her split P_1 would have kept projecting her negative component on the outside, on men in particular, preventing her from noticing others' appreciation of her. Thanks to the enactment in group, Eleonora was able to undertake a process of integration of her split parts that allowed her to curb her inner Persecutor's self-destructive nature. She finally started taking care of herself, adopting a healthier diet, with the help of a nutritionist, which led her to lose weight and cure the metabolic syndrome from which she had been suffering for several years.

The group changed too: it became more cohesive and intimate, and the differences between members, which had been smothered by the group's idealization of the therapist, are now more distinct. Everyone feels more at liberty to share the less socially acceptable parts of them.

In this clinical case we have seen how working with enactments within a group allowed Eleonora's traumatic past to emerge, with all its wounds, shame and dissociated relational units, but mostly, it allowed Eleonora to recognize her own hidden hopes and desires. Andrea, the new element in the group, represented that differentiated and differentiating Third (Benjamin, 2017), which broke down the symbiotic unity the therapist had maintained within the group for so long. "In my view, to see the client as solely a victim is a betrayal" claims (Little, 2016, p. 32). The therapist, caught in the shadow of the split together with Eleonora, had betrayed her, but in openly recognizing her betrayal she encouraged a more human behavior among members and stimulated everyone's collaboration. "The person who fails is paradoxically the one whom you desperately need to witness how she failed, to receive the communication" (Benjamin, 2017, p. 147).

To join clients in the abyss of repetition and then climb back up means opening up a space for past and present, old and new, and despair and hope: the paradoxical space of Thirdness.

Regressions toward more primitive personal interactions are, as we have seen in Chapter 4, precisely what gives the clients the opportunity to develop a more integrated self and more mature relationships, allowing the repeated elements to evolve into the needed relationship (Little, 2006). The group moved dialectically between script obligations and new forms of freedom. In this case, freedom is meant, on the one hand, as intra-psychic freedom, that is, the capacity to experience all ego states, even the ones buried for years under fear and shame; on the other hand, as freedom to verbally express oneself in unprecedented and spontaneous forms, involving affectively all group members. "As relational freedom expands . . . new unbidden meanings appear spontaneously, the way water rushes in to fill an empty space" (Stern, 2015, p. 116).

Transference and countertransference between dilution and intensification

While in individual therapy, the methods used by the therapist to deal with transference and countertransference dynamics are crucial to the treatment's success; in group therapy, the most important agents of change are the group itself and its cohesion.

According to Horwitz (1995), how the therapist processes the clients' transference within the group may contribute to alter the way transference is expressed among members. When the therapist assumes a neutral position, refusing to participate in games and emphasizing their leadership role, the group tends to regress and depend more and more on their leader. On the contrary, it is only when the therapist regards intersubjective dynamics and peer transferences as primary expressions, and not merely substitutes of the transferences projected onto them, that the group process is able to foster autonomy among its members. In such a case, the analysis of transference dynamics involves paying specific attention to the interpersonal learning happening between members. Transference analysis and interpersonal learning are both necessary in order for the clients to become capable of generalizing group experiences, extending them to life in the outside world: "Without this transfer or carryover, we have succeeded only in creating better, more gracious therapy group members" (Yalom & Leszcz, 2005, p. 292).

Horwitz (2018) identifies three elements specific to the group setting that are useful to dilute the intensity of the transference and, subsequently, to reduce paranoid, aggressive, fearful, or erotic feelings:

1   A decline of the idealizing transference: With respect to one-on-one sessions, in group, clients have a more comfortable relationship with the therapist; anxious reactions seem to be less intense, and clients, activating their Adult, have a more relaxed and constructive attitude.
2   A mitigation, thanks to the pressures of reality, of the client's fantasies to destroy or be destroyed by the therapist: The presence of other members

renders the situation more real, and, as a consequence, the therapist is perceived as less fearsome, which helps clients integrating their split P_1.

3   An increase of social and emotional distance: In group, the client has more opportunities to withdraw and take the role of the observer, gaining a better understanding of the games taking place.

However, beside forces contributing to a dilution of transference reactions, the group also contains forces which contribute to an intensification of these reactions.

The concordant and complementary identifications processes are at the basis of games within a group: when a member plays the role of the Victim, they may find Rescuers attuned to their problems and their need to be saved, but they may also spark complementary sadistic impulses.

Another reason behind the intensification of transference is the clients' frustration caused by the presence of other members, with whom they must share the therapist's time and attention. Each of them has the unpleasant feeling of not being unique and may either respond with explicit anxiety, envy, greed, and narcissism, or passively adapt and remain in the shadows, mulling over their frustration in their mind.

> Luca, a 26-year-old young man suffering from spastic-dystonic quadriplegia, arrives late to the fourth group session and starts talking right away about his anxiety, interrupting Elena, who was talking about her conflictual relationship with her abandoning mother. His lateness is caused by a medical appointment in which the doctors suggested the last in a series of painful operations on his right wrist tendon, in an attempt to improve mobility. Words come crashing out of his mouth, the others can barely understand what he is saying, his neck is stiff and his head, tilted up, twitches violently, but Luca does not seem to care. His only need is to release the deep frustration in the pit of his stomach: the frustration of being different, of having to undergo a constant stream of surgeries which cause him atrocious suffering, and of not being able to drive his wheelchair autonomously anymore. Elena, on the other hand, cannot accept the idea of someone taking away the space she fought for since the beginning of group treatment, and gets angry with him calling him selfish: "You only see your problems, you don't listen to us, your disability doesn't grant you permission to rob other people of their space!" While she says these words, she is gesturing wildly with her hands, but the rest of her body is stiff; she points her finger at Luca, like an angry teacher reprimanding a student who has done something irredeemable.

These words feel like a slap to Luca, who seems to finally awake from a trance: he will not let a fellow group member put him a corner. Now, he is looking straight at her; his deep eyes sharp as daggers. His stare fixed on her, his neck relaxed, his speech clear and precise, he says he feels like Elena failed to understand and listen to him in a moment of profound vulnerability, and goes on saying that he would have never expected to be treated so condescendingly by someone like her, who appeared sensitive and affectionate in the three previous sessions. Luca's anger restores dignity to his feeling of being different and to his desperate need to see himself as person like any other.

Luca and Elena's anger hide the fear that space – being a limited resource within the group – might be used up by others at their expense, leaving them to fight a battle for recognition. Elena did not treat Luca as if he was "different," but as an effective interlocutor to which assign boundaries. They are both prisoners of their wounds – Elena was abandoned by her mother, and Luca, whose parents are loving and caring, is being abandoned by a body that is leading him, slowly but inexorably, toward an almost complete immobility – and both of them are fighting to express the unbearableness of the injustices inflicted on them. This is the first step to reach one of the goals of group psychotherapy: accepting the differences between members by recognizing their similarities. Fellow members take care of Elena's and Luca's Child by trying to contain their intense emotions, almost tentatively, in the beginning, fearing to hurt one or the other, as if they felt the need to pick a side. After the therapists encourage members to talk about their own experiences in relation to what is happening with Elena and Luca, they share their need to feel unique, their fear of not being given the necessary amount of space, their shame related to the feeling of being invisible in the eyes of others. The fear and shame expressed by fellow members represent Elena's and Luca's dissociated parts: they both gave up their vulnerability to defend themselves from a threatening and abandonic world. The relationship conflict says something important about their inner relational units: the Persecutor Parent silences the Victim Child, who is afraid and full of shame (Little, 2006).

The therapists, faced with the first aggressive exchanges between Elena and Luca, are worried about the intensity of the feelings which, since the very first sessions, are emerging within the group, but they let members go through this experience together.[1] Thanks to the dilution of the transference, which granted them enough time to observe both games between members and their own countertransference reactions, they intervene legitimizing the work done by the group, which involved a deep struggle to recognize the other as separate subject, with similar but also different needs, a struggle they would have encountered again and again in subsequent group experiences. Tolerating this struggle is at the basis of group therapy.

It is impossible for Elena and Luca to get their needs entirely met, since, as Cornell and Bonds-White (2001) remind us, the therapeutic relationship does not revolve around gratification of the archaic desires of a client's Child. In group, repeated relationships have different outcomes than in the past, new experiences come to the surface and are made explicit and legitimized, and what before seemed irreconcilable – everyone's individual truths and needs – finds a new space where, from the old game of "You or Me," they can move on to the "Both you and me," meaning the space of the needed relationship in which past and present coexist within the group setting.

The work done in group consisted in an endless negotiation between Elena's and Luca's needs, first of all their need to be recognized. Recognition is something to be negotiated over and over because to be recognized is to recognize, to decentralize oneself, to relocate from oneself in order to open up to the other, and saying new words or expressing emotions never expressed before might mean to be disavowed by the group. It is a relationship negotiation which at times precedes, at times follows the negotiation of the inner spaces: the Adult, Child, and Parent parts, some known, some unknown, revealing their complexity and an absence of linearity.

The anxiety and anger of the first few sessions also represent the first shared group experience. All (including the therapists) step into the unknown with their own inner fantasies and script mechanisms. The sharing of anxieties and intense frustrations represents the first opportunity for group members to feel involved with each other and less isolated, which is the first step toward a group cohesion based on experience.

The group becomes a mother who is capable to see herself in and syntonize herself with her children's anger and jealousy, acting as regulator of the most intense emotional states, lowering the members' dissociative defenses.

The intensification of transference as described in the aforementioned clinical case recalled past experiences related to dysfunctional emotional states such as anger, shame, pain, and abandonment.

The dilution of countertransference, on the other hand, allowed the therapists to join in the clients' games and, at the same time, to reflect on the emotional components stirred up in them by the group: an emotionally taxing event fails to lead to any change in the group's life if the emotion is left unexamined by critical thought. When therapists have enough leeway to notice interruptions and obstacles in group communication, clients have in turn more freedom to move and contain into their minds all the different aspects of communication.

Countertransference as assessment tool

The therapist's countertransference is important in order to understand and process enactments. For this reason, we believe it necessary to understand the link between clinicians' emotional responses and clients' personality disorders. Kernberg (1965) conceives countertransference as the therapist's conscious emotional reaction to the clients' past experiences, and regards it as an important diagnostic tool.

Novellino considers the therapist's countertransference response as a crucial factor in helping the latter understand the ongoing relationship with their client and to strengthen the therapeutic alliance between the two (Novellino, 2004). The author compiled a list of questions useful to better understand the therapist's countertransference and use it in diagnostic terms (p. 139):

- Who does this client remind me of?
- Which unsatisfied need am I ascribing to them?
- Which ideal parental figure do they remind me of or do I wish they would be?
- Who talked like that?
- With whom have I ever felt similar feelings and emotions?
- With whom have I ever acted this way?
- Which role does my script provide for me when it comes to my professional life?
- Which role does the client play in my script?
- Which role do I play in the client's script?

These questions allow us to access the relational and intersubjective dimension of the therapeutic experience.

Colli and colleagues (Colli, Tanzilli, Dimaggio, & Lingiardi, 2014) conducted a study to further investigate such associations, and in Table 13.1, we have tried to integrate the results emerged from this inquiry by adding the other group members' possible reactions. In the following, we suggest a description at the social and functional level of the internal dialogue between the clinician's and group members' ego states, in order to highlight the behavior related to it and better understand which ego state is in control of the emotions, thoughts, and behaviors of the people in question.

Table 13.1 Patient's personality disorder, therapist's countertransference and transference between peers.

Personality disorders	Description of the therapist's countertransference responses	Description of transference between peers
Paranoid	Clinicians tend to activate their Adapted Child. They are afraid to say the wrong thing, to confront the client openly on their contradictions or their exasperating behaviors; in fear, they might decide to leave or have a violent reaction. In other moments, therapists activate their Critical Parent, experiencing anger and hostility toward the client.	On a social level, members manifest a fear of facing the client's anger, but, on a psychological level, they wish the latter would leave, fantasizing that the therapist kick them out, finally freeing members from the "disturbance."
Schizoid	Therapists feel inadequate and incompetent, and often activate their Adapted Child. They have some trouble establishing a therapeutic alliance with the client.	Other members experience the client as someone too different from them, so they feel a strong sense of distance and feel rejected every time they try to get closer to them.
Schizotypical	Clinicians tend to activate their Critical Parent; they are annoyed, distracted, and irritated by this client.	When a client suffering from this disorder talks about themselves, other members tend to look at the clock impatiently, their mind is elsewhere, their Child feels like they are sitting in a classroom at school, listening to a boring lesson.
Borderline	The clinicians' main driver with these clients is "Try Hard." They try hard when they activate their fearful Child, when they feel responsible for a client's relapse and when they feel "forced" to prolong a session or grant extra phone calls.	Members fluctuate between the Adapted Child, as the therapist, and the angry Child, because they perceive the client as "special" in the eyes of the therapist. There are also moments, however, in which they mobilize their Adult, as when they give feedback to the client in order to pull them back to an appropriate reality testing. In such cases, members are able to contact the importance they hold for this client during the latter's moments of stability.
Histrionic	Therapists are rather involved with these clients; they let themselves feel all the emotions, at times activating their Free Child and ending up revealing their opinions or some aspects of their personal lives.	Group members are very active with regard to this client; they are involved in the latter's emotional intensity and they feel driven to share with them some deep parts of themselves. On a psychological level, sometimes members perceive the histrionic client as too exasperating and dramatic, experiencing anger at being excluded from this kind of relationship with the therapist.

Narcissistic	Therapists oscillate between irritation, boredom, and the need to feel admired and esteemed. Their Adapted Child feels useless, invisible, and incapable, while their Parent swings between the roles of Rescuer and Persecutor.	The most adapted group members benefit from this client because in part, they can identify with aspects of their selfishness and in part they feel driven to intervene in an assertive manner against the client's greed. More assertive members, on the other hand, mobilize their Critical Parent and their Adult, tending to confront the client openly.
Avoidant	Clinicians tend to mobilize their Nurturing Parent and take care of this client, containing the latter's anxieties and fears. During the therapeutic process, therapists activate their Critical Parent in relation to the client's family, which has been unable to fulfill the client's emotional needs. When it comes to this client, therapists are hopeful for a positive outcome to the treatment.	The avoidant client attracts the sympathy of their fellow group members, who, as the therapist, are very protective toward them and attribute them an important aggregating function. Members miss this client when they are absent and pay special attention to their contributions.
Dependent	With this client, too, therapists activate their Nurturing Parent. They feel the need to offer the client what others could not or would not give them. With them, as with the histrionic client, during sessions therapists tend to talk about themselves a lot and reveal much more than with other clients. Other times, on the contrary, they might feel bored or helpless, but mostly frustrated by the slow pace at which change happens in clients such as this.	Thanks to their tendency to please others, the dependent client earns all fellow members' approval. This client always pay attention to members' problems and they often come to members' rescue with interesting or useful arguments. However, to members, this client comes across as boring when they talk about themselves, because they lack spontaneity and intimacy.
Obsessive-Compulsive	Clinicians often experience feelings of boredom, withdrawal, and irritation. They do not regard working with obsessive-compulsive clients as compelling and they tend not to talk about themselves when supervising.	The presence of obsessive-compulsive clients in the group is tolerated but not appreciated by fellow members. The latter get bored listening to the client's hyper-detailed and stereotyped description of themselves. Members who tend to adapt withdraw in their own silence, more assertive members, instead, tend to interrupt the obsessive-compulsive client, openly manifesting their boredom.

Source: Adapted from Colli et al. (2014)

Conclusions

During group sessions, Berne used to have trainees sit in a circle outside the clients' circle and, 20 minutes before the end of therapy, trainees switched places with clients, who listened to the trainees' reflections on the dynamics observed up until that moment and could interact with trainees themselves (Berne, 1968). In this communicative and meditative exchange, we can make out Berne's intention to recognize clients as active and constructive participants of the therapeutic process.

Relational transactional analysts have built on this intention by electing to see countertransference as a tool allowing them to understand in the here-and-now of therapy the there-and-then of clients. But the here-and-now is not merely a reprise of the script: it is a meeting place, a vivid scenario in which conflicts are reintroduced under a new light, because the subjects involved are different. In this context, the therapist creates a relational space in which the transference–countertransference matrix "plays" an important role. Playing in the therapy room is akin to be a child again, when the meaning of the game was established by one's ability to coordinate with others, co-create rules and rhythms: when somebody in the group stubbornly refused to accept the rules, the game would stop. Working within the transference–countertransference matrix and, above all, working with enactments is similar to intensely reexperiencing that rupture of shared rhythm and rules. Games become part of the interactions entangled in the intersubjective field: not only do they represent a powerful mode of unconscious communication, but, through the therapist's nurturing tolerance, they also become an important tool for affect regulation. Such relational impasses lead both clients and therapist to interrupt a work characterized by rules and shared goals, to find themselves angry and wounded antagonists, or, in other scenarios, accomplices in an atmosphere of defeat and hopelessness, as we has seen happen in the case of Eleonora. With games, group therapy stops pursuing the goal of making script mechanisms visible any longer; instead, it seeks the transformation and integration of the ego states through the emotional regulation of dissociated mental/cerebral areas.

Note

1 After the end of the session, comparing their perspectives on the events, both therapists agreed that their silence was facilitated by the fact that they were not alone in leading the group. The trust each therapist put into the other allowed both of them to surrender to group regression, at the same time harboring the hope that all group members would have benefited from this moment of rupture but also profound authenticity.

References

Benjamin, J. (2017). *Beyond doer and done to: Recognition theory, intersubjectivity and the third.* London and New York: Routledge, Taylor & Francis Group.

Berne, E. (1964). *Games people play: The psychology of human relationships.* New York: Grove Press.

Berne, E. (1968). Staff-patient staff conferences. *American Journal of Psychiatry*, *125*(3), 286–293. doi:10.1176/ajp.125.3.286

Bucci, W. (1997). *Psychoanalysis and cognitive science: A multiple code theory*. New York: Guilford Press.

Chang, V., & James, M. (1987). Anxiety and projection as related to games and scripts. *Transactional Analysis Journal*, *17*(4), 178–184. doi:10.1177/036215378701700408

Colli, A., Tanzilli, A., Dimaggio, G., & Lingiardi, V. (2014). Patient personality and therapist response: An empirical investigation. *The American Journal of Psychiatry*, *171*(1), 102–108. doi:10.1176/appi.ajp.2013.13020224

Cornell, W. F., & Bonds-White, F. (2001). Therapeutic relatedness in transactional analysis: The truth of love or the love of truth. *Transactional Analysis Journal*, *31*(1), 71–83. doi:10.1177/036215370103100108

Edelman, G. M. (1989). *The remembered present: A biological theory of consciousness*. New York: Basic Books.

Horwitz, L. (1995). Discussion of "group as a whole". *International Journal of Group Psychotherapy*, *45*(2), 143–148. doi:10.1080/00207284.1995.11490767

Horwitz, L. (2018). *Listening with the fourth ear: Unconscious dynamics in analytic group psychotherapy*. New York: Routledge.

Jacobs, T. J. (1986). On countertransference enactments. *Journal of the American Psychoanalytic Association*, *34*(2), 289–307. doi:10.1177/000306518603400203

Karpman, S. (1968). Fairy tales and script drama analysis. *Transactional Analysis Bulletin*, *7*(26), 9–43. Retrieved from https://karpmandramatriangle.com/pdf/DramaTriangle.pdf

Kernberg, O. (1965). Notes on countertransference. *Journal of the American Psychoanalytic Association*, *13*(1), 38–56. doi:10.1177/000306516501300102

Lingiardi, V., & McWilliams, N. (Eds.). (2017). *Psychodynamic diagnostic manual: PDM-2* (2nd ed.). New York: The Guilford Press.

Little, R. (2006). Ego state relational units and resistance to change. *Transactional Analysis Journal*, *36*(1), 7–19. doi:10.1177/036215370603600103

Little, R. (2016). Transference-countertransference focused transactional analysis. In R. G. Erskine (Ed.), *Transactional analysis in contemporary psychotherapy* (1st ed., pp. 27–53). London: Routledge. doi:10.4324/9780429484179

Novak, E. T. (2015). Are games, enactments, and reenactments similar? No, yes, it depends. *Transactional Analysis Journal*, *45*(2), 117–127. doi:10.1177/0362153715578840

Novellino, M. (2004). *Psicoanalisi transazionale*. Milano: Franco Angeli.

Schore, A. N. (2020). Forging connections in group psychotherapy through right brain-to-right brain emotional communications. Part 1: Theoretical models of right brain therapeutic action. Part 2: Clinical case analyses of group right brain regressive enactments. *International Journal of Group Psychotherapy*, *70*(1), 29–88. doi:10.1080/00207284.2019.1682460

Stern, D. B. (2015). *Relational freedom: Emergent properties of the interpersonal field*. New York: Routledge Taylor & Francis Group.

Stuthridge, J. (2015). All the world's a stage: Games, enactment, and countertransference. *Transactional Analysis Journal*, *45*(2), 104–116. doi:10.1177/0362153715581174

Yalom, I. D., & Leszcz, M. (2005). *The theory and practice of group psychotherapy* (5th ed.). New York: Basic Books (Original work published 1970).

14

DREAMWORK IN GROUP THERAPY

Dreams and groups have always been connected, both in literature and in the psychoanalytic experience, from Foulkes (1964) to Bion (1992) to the more recent studies of Neri, Pines, and Friedman (2002). The group's atmosphere is considered oneiric on its own because of the powerful regressive effect the group spontaneously induces in clients. A little like taking a group of adults in suit and tie back to the experience of sitting around a prehistoric fire, barefoot, and dressed in animal leathers.

In group, dreams create a common sense, increase emotional connections between members, facilitate the expression of up until that moment unverbalized emotions, and prepare to problem solving and the healing experience.

According to Winnicott (1971), the oneiric work takes place in what he defines the third intermediate area of experience, the in-between, the space of curiosity, exploration, and discovery: a playground.

Dreams are an effort of the self to restore its psychic structure, and in group, the listener must stay close to the dreamer in empathic syntonization, without entering the game of interpretation or looking for any real meaning.

Among recent psychoanalytic studies, we find Wilma Bucci's (1997) studies on the multiple code particularly useful to understand the goal of dreamwork in group, which is to reconnect the split parts of our clients' body-mind in order to strengthen referential ability and integration of the self. The definitions of healthy and pathological referential cycles also include the answers to the question of what use we should make of dreams and groups in psychotherapy:

> In the first stage of the cycle, the patient may experience diverse nonverbal components of the emotion schemas, including specific sub-symbolic elements – feelings, smells, bodily experience, action patterns – which he has difficulty expressing directly in words. In the second phase, the patient may retrieve a specific memory or fantasy derived from past experience, events of the day, or events in the treatment relationship; here, the connection of the subsymbolic contents to images and then to words is made. Optimally, in the third phase, the patient reflects upon the images and stories that have been told, and further connections within

DOI: 10.4324/9781003215547-15

the verbal system and in the shared discourse may be made. Ultimately, the process of verbalizing the contents of the emotion schemas lays the foundation for labeling the emotion itself: "I feel rage"; "I am afraid." The new connections within the verbal and non-verbal system then may feed back to open the emotion schemas further, thus continuing the cycle on a deeper level.

A progression of this nature may also be traced in the construction and interpretation of dreams. The latent contents, primarily in sub-symbolic format, are connected to the discrete specific images of the manifest contents, which are then verbalized in the dream narrative (Bucci, 1993; Bucci, Severino, & Creelman, 1991). In the interpretation of the dream, the latent contents, including wishes and other emotion structures that have been warded off, may eventually themselves be acknowledged and verbalized.

The development of emotional meaning in free association and dreams has its roots in the basic processes of emotional development itself. Normal emotional development depends on the integration of somatic, sensory, and motoric processes in the emotion schemas; emotional disorders are caused by failure of this integration.

(Bucci, 1997, p. 160)

Our model of dream analysis in group is explorative, focusing on the creative process of the dream and the co-creation of the discussion on dreams in the group environment. Here, in particular, we will describe dreams that have been narrated and analyzed in group settings, in which the work is centered on the analysis of the group imago and how this imago, through deconfusion and healing processes, changes and distances itself from the script themes, enriching the clients' inner and interpersonal world with new reparative and integrative experiences.

A transactional analysis approach on dreams

Berne (1957) wrote, "It is probable also that dreams have another function, and that is to assist in healing the mind after emotional wounds and distressing emotional experiences" (p. 16). In transactional analysis, we might say that it is the dreamer who writes the script. By this, I mean that the dream is constructed predominantly in the language of the Child ego state, in accordance with the logic, emotive intensity, and decisional choices of the Little Professor (the precursor of the Adult ego state or A_1). This is the state of mind that decides the psychological script. Thus, in this sense, access to dreams is fundamental for the discovery of the unconscious parts of the script and for revealing to both client and therapist how this Child mind works and has so much power over survival choices and emotional decisions.

Literature on dream analysis in TA has seen many contributions, from Berne to many representatives of redecision therapy. From the 2000s, Bowater (1999, 2001, 2003, 2008, 2009, 2010, 2013) and Bowater and Sherrard (2011) provided major contributions on dream analysis, comparing the transactional analytic experience with the most recent studies on dreams, in both the neuroscientific and psychodynamic field.

The theme of the "script dream," which was introduced by Berne in *What Do You Say After You Say Hello?* (1972, pp. 172–175), clarifies the psychodynamic perspective from which our observation starts. The script dream has nothing to do with the client's real life but, rather, uses a figurative image to describe the close limits within which a person is confined by script decisions. The "concentration camp" or the patient's "tunnel," as cited by Berne, will explain to the therapist why certain clients improve but do not heal unless these limits are overcome. Bowater (2013) described a client's repetitive nightmares as script dreams and how the attribution of meaning to the nightmare affords some clients sufficient awareness to come out of the script tunnel.

Dreams in the different developmental stages of the group

Therapy work in the Bernian group is centered on group imago analysis, which also features, through a close look at its evolution, in a client's process of deconfusion.

We have seen how dream narration in group changes according to the evolutionary stages of group imago (Clarkson, 1992):

During the first stage, people have a provisional imago and projections that emerge in dreams are related to the client's script themes. It is as if the client presented themselves to others in a symbolic fashion, with their own insignia, armor, and their family's colors, just like a medieval knight, and expressed their courage (this is who I am), but also their fear of entering in foreign territory such as that of the group.

In a second stage, that of the temporarily adapted group imago, what emerges are dreams about conflict and the monsters that used to dominate the world of the Child writing the script.

In a third stage, that of the operative group imago, dreams contain ambivalent group situations, at times terrifying, at times protective.

In the fourth stage, especially, dreams explicitly feature the therapist, other group members, and collective situations in which the group is strongly symbolized as a healing force. In the fourth stage, dreams anticipate the healing process, the emergence of the client's curative internal forces and their fears about the future.

Toward the end of the process and after the end of therapy, dreams contain elements of sadness, but also representations of a parental blessing for a new departure from home, this time as a more mature and adult individual.

Usually, the role other members play in dreams is extraordinarily rich of valuable intuitions on each member's script. It is not incidental that somebody appears in dreams as a fellow adventurer, someone else as a seducer, others as persecutors, and so on.

Through dreams, each client's Child plays "pretend," dresses themselves and others up for theatrical representations which reveal script scenes and even protocol, archaic scenes which generated the emotional backdrop of the script decisions. Sharing the dream, narrating it to others and "playing" at interpreting it is even more interesting.

The therapist thinks: What is this person telling us though the dream?
In his text *Man and His Symbols*, Jung says:

> Thus a word or an image is symbolic when it implies something more than its obvious and immediate meaning. It has a wider "unconscious" aspect. . . . As the mind explores the symbol, it is led to ideas that lie beyond the grasp of reason.
> (Jung, Franz, Henderson, Jaffé, & Jacobi, 1964, pp. 20–21)

Narrated dreams in psychotherapy groups

Through the actions and feelings clients manifest in group, the experience, or protocol, that formed the basis of their script decisions is rapidly and clearly revealed. It is visible in transference toward the therapist, other group members, and the group itself. Added to the communicative behaviors observable by the therapist are the narrations of the clients, who present an account of themselves that is usually different from and complementary to the one the therapist has heard in individual sessions. To these narrations of the client's past history and present life are eventually added the narration of dreams.

Phase 1: Provisional group imago

Through the dream I am telling you who I am and what I am afraid of.
Not all clients bring up their dreams in the first stage of the group. Some had dreams before joining the group, but it often happens that they are revealed to the group only after a while. Those who bring their dreams to the group from the very beginning often use them as self-introduction tools. When employed this way, dreams are characterized by dramatic and spectacular traits, often charged with references to the script.

Irene's dream

Irene is a 35-year-old woman who embarks on therapy in a period of depression brought on by the end of a partnership and a change of city and job. She is beginning to live alone after her entire life has fallen apart with the end of her relationship. She describes her dream:

I'm at your [the therapist's] house, there are a lot of people, and I go up to you. Some purebred fighting dogs are arriving. You've

---

let them come in! I say to you, "What the hell are you doing?"
I put out my arm to protect myself and one of the dogs bites me.
I think: He did it out of revenge because I had hit you lightly. I am
resigned to the fact that the dog will always bite me. I won't be
able to free myself; he'll drag me along, and I'll have to follow
him. The entrance door seems to be made of cardboard. There are
some Arabs outside who are trying to get in, and I wake up feeling
anguish.

In the group analysis of Irene's dream, she says, "I know I'm afraid of the group, and I feel very aggressive toward the others at the same time." A member of the group adds, "Often you seem as if you might bite when you speak, your remarks are very cutting." Irene recognizes the truth of this and offers, "Actually, I'm afraid of being bitten in my turn and that the therapist won't protect me, leaving me alone to be dragged along by my anger, the mastiff."

Out of the group discussion another meaning also emerges: the dog that bites her is also the recurrence of depression and dysphoria. After this dream Irene feels more at ease in the group.

Irene then has a second dream related to the group, which she describes as follows:

There's a child who doesn't resemble me, a boy, accompanied by a
woman. He sits down to have a pair of roller skates put on. Then
a man, who is my father, says: "Speak, Speak." And the woman
says, "Can't you see that he has lost his speech? He has to get used
to his new condition." And then I say, "Try roller blades, they're
faster!"

In the next group, Irene explains,

For me, falling into depression is like losing my speech: To avoid having to feel, I run around doing lots of things. I don't have the words to say how I feel. I feel like a child, not a woman. For me, it's difficult to sit for 2 hours listening to you. I try not to stop at all, as if I were on skates.

Some in the group observe, "It's true, we can see that at times you'd like to get away from us."

During a psychodynamic therapy, dreams are always moments of intense communication between client and therapist. When a client starts remembering their dreams and bringing them up in therapy, they are trying to communicate something important to themselves and the therapist through the cryptic and dense language of dreams.

In the logic of the treatment we are describing, a dream is a message the client sends themselves, and the help they ask the therapist is in decoding the message itself, which sometimes can appear incomprehensible, even though often accompanied by strong emotions, more frequently distressing and hardly ever pleasant. In group, dreams are also an important way to symbolically tell something about oneself to fellow group members: I am telling you what I am afraid of, I am shocking you with strong images, I want to inspire fear in you, or I want to invite you to get close to me.

Those who listen to the dream (therapist and group members) find themselves in the same position as the archaeologist faced with the ruins of a pyramid in the desert. The approach to this world of symbols and broken memories belonging to somebody we do not know must be gentle, and it is the therapist's responsibility to facilitate a climate of non-judgmental listening in group.

Thus, the appropriate attitude when listening to a dream is exploration.

Furthermore, we need to be aware of the fact that we are faced with a language rich in images and thus, as with a painting or, even better, a surreal movie, there is not just one interpretation, meaning that we cannot expect the dream to follow a linear second-order logic.

An image evokes, contains within itself the power to recall emotions and multiple meanings: we are closer to the symbol than narration. Thus, symbolic and "figurative" language, poetic density, metaphor, and analogy: This is the alphabet of the oneiric world. A Child language, often forgotten and become inaccessible to the Adult, who is no longer able to grasp right away the message coming from within.

Berne (1957) wrote:

> It is a common error to suppose that finding out the meaning of the dream is the important thing. This is not so. The meanings must be felt, and these feelings must be put into proper perspective with other past and present feelings of that particular person, for the interpretation to have any effect in changing the underlying Id tensions, which is the purpose of the procedure.
>
> (pp. 136–137)

The usefulness of dreamwork in therapy is in leading the client to face emotions and contents that upset them, and helping them become familiar with their inner monsters, as well as learn how to listen to their inner advisor (the Little Professor), who is trying to survive as best as they can. But during a psychodynamic therapy, the dream is also, in particular, an extension of script analysis: As if the client, having just come out of a group or individual session, kept working to find a new balance, trying, through trial and error, to re-decide their script system.

If the therapist believes that the client has activated a little, intuitive inner therapist within themselves, working in dreams to find solutions and solve enigmas, therapist and client will be able to find a valid nocturnal help to the diurnal work of analysis. The dreamer is the nocturnal researcher working in alliance with us, and thus a valuable and unique collaborator to the process of understanding and change the client's desires, however scared this change makes them.

Phase 2: Adapted imago – The conflict

Conflict is also represented in the oneiric work, to both therapist and group, in indirect ways, through forms of masking which often imply strongly distressing contents. At a later stage, while moving from the temporarily adapted imago to the operative imago (where games come into play), the emerging dreams feature conflicts and the same monsters which dominated the world of the Child writing the script.

Bet's dreams

Bet is a 27-year-old phobic woman with an anxiety problem and various psychosomatic illnesses. She has difficulty speaking at work, tends to isolate herself, and finds it difficult to defend her rights and face up to others. Her illnesses include irritable bowel syndrome and a serious case of bruxism (for which she must wear a shield) that causes jaw pain, especially at night. Her difficulty in speaking and facing others also manifests in group. After a year, she reports this dream:

> I feel a strong sensation of helplessness. I want to open my mouth but it won't open. The upper part of my mouth and my upper jaw sink into my lower teeth. The bottom right canine feels wobbly and falls out, like a milk tooth. The canine has a hole in it. It's hollow because it has been crushed by the top teeth. I continue to destroy the molars too, and they flake. Oh my god, what am I doing? I was scared, but my upper jaw seemed to be automatic, out of control. It was like a ceiling falling on top of me.

Bet said about the dream: The strange thing is that when I woke up, I didn't have any muscle pain. But from then on I've had jaw and neck pain.

Bet's jaw pain, nocturnal contraction of the mouth, and teeth grinding began at age 15. She says that her upper jaw represents her ability to control things, to reveal nothing, to keep to herself. To remain silent about her secrets, to tell lies, and not to speak about herself to others is important to her as a way of avoiding the judgment of others, which she greatly fears. "I've always felt judged by my father, always in the wrong in his eyes. If I don't say anything about myself, I avoid being judged." She adds that she greatly fears aggression in others, that she does not know how to defend herself except by walking away. To her, the hollow canine, like a milk tooth, represents this difficulty in "using her teeth," that is, in showing the aggressiveness that is sometimes useful, especially at work.

After sharing and talking about this dream in group, Bet took a more active part in group conversations. She revealed her emotions and trained herself to be assertive at work and also in group as observed by other group members.

Phase 3: Operative imago

When group members start dreaming explicitly about the group and fellow members, we are at a deep stage of the analytical work: transactions go beyond pastimes and divided themselves in games, activities, and intimacy. The internalization of the group experience involves a representation of the group itself in the oneiric scenario, which often includes a manifest rechilding process with the introduction of new environments and contents in the client's oneiric life. It is particularly interesting, in this phase, to analyze the association processes taking place in the "interchange of oneiric material" with other members.

The whole group dreams about the group

The context in which the dreams described here take place is a therapy group of women in their thirties plus one around 50. We heard about these dreams during the therapy group itself.

Giusi is a 30-year-old woman whose studies are at a standstill because of recurring depression, although she is close to graduating. Terry is a 50-year-old woman, the mother of two children, in therapy for the difficulties that she has in close relationships and for her tendency to isolate herself. This is Giusi's dream:

I was waiting for Terry in a house; she was in a hurry and had to transfer some wine into a large demijohn. She was in a rush and said she didn't have time for a coffee. I go into another room and get a text message from you [the therapist] with some joyful symbols, and we interpret them. The expected twins have been born. [Giusi goes on to say that she associates this image with the entrance of two men in the group after a long period of only women.]

Maria is a 32-year-old physiotherapist in treatment for difficulties in establishing close relationships. She recounts her dream:

I was in a group with you two [cotherapists] and two others. We were at your house [she turns to one of the therapists]. There was a narrow corridor, a lot of books and armchairs. I'm speaking and you get a phone call from a client that makes you really angry. You're really harsh and slam the phone down on him. I finish speaking about my feeling of loneliness. You ask me something else, and I start crying. I can see darkness, you come up to me and hug me. I wake up with a feeling of well-being from the hug.

Maria commented,

I feel more open toward love. I feel different. I feel that there's less distance between you and me. The other week I dreamed that I had to go to bed with a really old oriental guru, and now I'm able to let myself be hugged in the group.

Bianca is a 28-year-old woman who suffers from anxiety and food disorders. She graduated from university after an interruption in her studies. She tells us the following dream:

I was supposed to come for group therapy, and I find myself in a group of strangers, in a place I don't know. I hear they are speaking about sex education, and I feel incredibly uneasy. At the end of this hour, I have to come here, and I ask someone for information. It's you, and I pay you for the hour of sex education. I feel really anxious. I was at a party; it was a big space, and I had the feeling that I'd done something wrong [feeling of guilt]. There were faces I didn't recognize that showed disapproval of me. I argued violently with someone, and then I ran off. I came away by myself. I went into a house and picked up a cushion. I climbed out of the window really upset. I was upset, it was raining, I had the cushion

with me, and I was crying. I got to your house [the therapist's],
and there's a veranda full of black men eating. I ask after you, and
they tell me that you aren't in but to wait for you there. I sit down
with them and I feel relieved. I wait for you.

Bianca's comment about the dream was that "it came after a week of nocturnal nightmares, agitation, and sweating." She is exploring her sexuality
and through the group has been experiencing an education in sex that goes
against the injunctions "Do not enjoy it" and "Don't be close."

Kati is a 35-year-old woman who is in therapy because she is not satisfied
with her close relationships and does not seem able to have children. Her
dream is as follows:

We are at a special group session at my family home, which turns
out to be the therapist's house. I express my need for attention to
the therapist, who hugs me and strokes me for a long time. I'm
pleasantly disturbed by it. She continues to stroke me for so long
that I begin to think the others might be jealous. When everyone
has gone, I remain with the therapist and tell her that I've had a
dream that I'd like to tell her about, but she doesn't have time. She
has to go to a rugby match, but she says I can stay at her house
anyway. I'm alone, and my partner arrives; I tell him that this isn't
my house any longer, that it's the therapist's house and he can stay
there as well.

Kati noted that she was experiencing a conflict between her desire for a
new phase of individual therapy and her link to the group. The other group
participants point out that in the dream there is a representation of contact
and closeness that she does not usually show.

Terry, as described earlier, is a 50-year-old woman, the mother of two
children, in therapy for difficulties in her close relationships and a tendency
to isolate herself. She relates the following dream:

We are guests, my theater group and I, in an apartment, and we
have to act out our show there. I'm pregnant and sleep in a room
with another girl. The therapist and her husband come into the
apartment to see the show. I sit them down on a sofa and try to
turn on the television to entertain them. The husband appears to
be skeptical: How can I act if I'm pregnant? I shouldn't be doing
it. We haven't rehearsed it yet, there's no time. I'm afraid I won't
remember my lines, and I feel alone and unprepared.

Terry was effectively engaging in acting in her life, but the interesting aspect is the pregnancy, which is experienced by all the women participating in the group as a reminder of the change that is taking place within the group (two men come in, the twins dreamt of by Giusi) and also in the life of Terry (new decisions and greater willingness to become closer to the others).

Phase 4: Secondarily adjusted imago

Phase 4 discusses the representation of healing through the narration of the dream to the group. Psychotherapy should conclude with the achievement of the aims of the contract, hence with the solving of the problems that prompted the client to seek treatment and personal analysis. Both therapist and client have in mind an idea of how the therapy should conclude. It is important that these representations are explicitly stated and explored.

Healing for most people means growing, abandoning pretense and infantile illusions, and being able to stand on their own two feet in the adult world by means of their own strengths and with the help of others. It also means helping others in return, on the basis of reciprocity.

Berne (1966) wrote that

> the therapist should remember that while death is a tragedy, life is a comedy. (Furthermore, even one's own deaths not always a tragedy as such; it may only become tragic in its effects on others.) Curiously enough, many clients reverse this dramatic principle, and treat life like a tragedy and death like a comedy. The therapist who follows them is once more a party of a folie-à-deux.
>
> (p. 289)

Keith Tudor (Summers & Tudor, 2005), teacher of TA, would say that healing also means discovering our condition of We-ness, meaning what makes us human beings beyond the dual condition of you and I.

This research of the true self constitutes the objective of the analytical journey and thus healing means putting a client in the condition of being able to communicate with their true self, without having to give up the world and intimate relationships. Berne (1972) would say that therapy wants to make a prince out of a frog, and to do so it must "flip in" the client, taking them out of the script and into the real world. The script antithesis is a powerful message the therapist conveys whenever the client is ready to re-decide, to "flip in," to transform from client into "real person raring to go."

All this, according to Berne, can happen in a single dialectic exchange, and, might we add, only if in that moment the client is ready to accept the message with the necessary intensity for it to penetrate deeply and be kept within like a permission or a blessing.

The separation between therapist and client is an experience to live, analyze, elaborate, and, we could say, mentalize.[1]

The therapist must announce that this moment will come, it is fundamental they make the client imagine and anticipate it in order to discuss it together, to explore the multiple and often ambivalent feelings and thoughts it sparks.

Daniel J. Siegel, in his splendid book *The Developing Mind*, describes the strategies of collaborative communication which generate a secure attachment, and talks about the process of integration of minds as a process that allows growth and regeneration also through psychotherapeutic treatments.

If therapy works, writes Siegel (1999):

This new capacity for integration – both interpersonal and internal – may create a sense of vitality and a release of creative energy and ideas, leading to an invigorating sense of personal expression. Such spontaneous and energized processes can give rise to participation in various activities, such as painting, music, dance, poetry, creative writing, or sculpture. It can also yield a deeper sense of creativity and appreciation within the "everyday" experience of life: communication with others, walks down the street, new appreciation of the richness of perceptions, feelings of being connected to the flow of the moment (p. 335).

And adds: "It is in these heightened moments of engagement, these dyadic states of resonance, that one can appreciate the power of relationships to nurture and to heal the mind" (p. 337).

Giulio's dreams

Giulio is 28 years old when he starts therapy. He is a nurse and lives with his widowed mother. He is awkward in social relationships and unable to find a girlfriend. He was epileptic as a child and shows great anxiety when speaking in public. He interrupts himself and cannot finish his sentences. He dresses inadequately, often makes himself look ugly, and appears ill-tempered. I put him into a group after a few months of individual treatment, and we witness a good deal of improvement in his social and conversational abilities. The level of anxiety in his dreams rises.

Giulio's recurring nightmare is of a monster that he never sees but that leaves traces of killings. The monster frequently chases after him and the characters in his dreams. For 2 years, the monster terrorizes Giulio's nights. At a certain point in the analysis of his dreams, Giulio finally bursts into tears and says, "I fear that I'm the monster, I've always been afraid of becoming a serial killer, of being monstrous. Perhaps that's why I can't find a woman." Speaking to the women in the group proves extremely useful to

Giulio, helping him to realize that he makes himself appear ugly and that he has had an active role in getting himself rejected.

As Novellino (1998) suggested, it is important not to underestimate the psychodynamics of nightmares and the importance of correctly understanding how they reflect central, conflictual themes that arise during psychotherapy. After deeper analysis, the theme of the monster will be associated by Giulio to his epilepsy and the fears of losing control generated by the illness.

Later Giulio has a new dream:

> *I'm with some others of the group hunting the monster. I run toward a house we know he's gone into, we run together toward a central room where he's locked himself in. I force the door, and I'm astonished to see that the room is empty – it's light, with white walls, and the sun is streaming in through the windows.*

Here, Giulio starts crying, which is liberating and a relief for him. The dream provides a powerful image of the redecision he made during therapy. Not long after this, Giulio falls in love, marries, and ends his psychotherapy.

Phase 5: Clarified group imago – Farewells to therapist and group

"The converse of the script is the real person living in a real world" (Berne, 1972, p. 276).

The following message was sent to me by Giulia, who had finished group treatment some months before:

> *Hi. The other night I dreamed about you. Strange that in all the years of therapy I never dreamed about you, yet now that I'm out of the group, this is already the second time. When you appear, it's a really nice feeling, I'd say one of trust and recognition. This time, although I got out of bed to write down the dream, unfortunately I wasn't able to. Some time ago, I dreamed about my mum, with whom I was arguing about a wedding or something like that. Afterward, in the dream, you appear, and we're walking together, climbing up a spiral staircase. You speak a bit on the phone about some business of yours in front of me. You don't care if I hear you.*

148

Then the staircase leads to a big room, like the lobby of a hotel/ congress/exhibition (that's the impression I get), and we have a snack, talking to each other around a small, round, high table, like in a bar. I don't remember anything else, but I know that the bad feeling of the argument has changed into one of acceptance, of welcome and serenity.

Giulia had a long group therapy treatment for depression that had thrown obstacles in the path of her university studies and life. Now she works, lives with a partner, and has found her own equilibrium, although she has had to combat her Parent ego state's expectations of a perfect life that she felt incapable of fulfilling.

Fanny's dream

Fanny is 32 years old and a psychologist who is just finishing her group therapy. She is processing her grief at the end of therapy, which coincides with her leaving the family home. She reports the following dream:

I'm at [redacted]. I go to the place where I have therapy to share the joys and emotions of the conference [the success of a public intervention of hers]. When I get there, I find it's very dark. It's an immense loft overlooking a port. The building is dilapidated. I see that the therapist is all energy, and I don't want to be seen. I'm scared that she thinks I'm in the way. I sit beside Ilaria, who is working and doesn't pay any attention to me. Then Andrea arrives and gives me a guided tour. There's a corner all of glass, and I look out of the window. The sky is grey, and the water of the port is sluggish and putrid. On a terrace I see a lot of old desks lined up, and I think how weatherbeaten they are. On one of them there's the therapist's bag. Andrea takes me into a corridor, and I realize that it's made up of old and new tiles, all side by side and all different. I ask why it's such a mosaic, and he answers that new tiles have been put in where there were missing ones, but that those that were there have been kept in place. I think that it's a shoddy job, but Andrea shrugs his shoulders and doesn't agree with me.

Fanny is in the process of finding a house of her own, and she has a new job. She must reconcile the conflicting emotions linked to so many changes, the old and the new tiles, her pleasure at her new life and her sadness at having to say farewell.

A summary of the therapy in one of Aldo's dreams recounted toward the end of group therapy

First scene: I'm in car parked near a beach and a river (sunset). The sea is agitated, there's a lot of wind, there's a storm coming. I'm sitting in the car, looking out. People are scared, the tension is high. I tell myself: I need to leave!

Emotions associated with the first scene: Annoyance, worry. It's the situation I was in when I started therapy: I was alone in the middle of a storm, what was happening and what I was causing was dangerous.

Second scene: I'm on a treadmill with many people. I'm with E., my 10-year-old daughter. There's a narrowing, an obstacle: We need to get past it without getting off the treadmill. I'm telling my little girl: Let's hold hands with a stranger.

Emotions associated with the second scene: Surprise for having trusted a stranger with my daughter. I think it's the group experience that's like a treadmill, where you take strangers by the hand and you feel protected by this contact with them.

Third scene: I find myself in a house made out of stone. I know I have to go in, the stairs are full of thorny brambles. In the garden, I can see my dad and my friend Vittorio looking at me. I climb the stairs and when I turn around I see a giant bear in the garden.

Emotions associated with the third scene: Physical sensations to my hands, as if I was moving the brambles' branches to climb the stairs; surprise because of the bear; I feel like I am the bear and the house of stone; satisfaction to see my dad and my friend there to support me. I'm finding myself once again.

Aldo came to therapy because he wanted to kill his wife's lover. He had a terrible explosion of rage and was stopped one night by his friend Vittorio (present in the third scene of the dream), who kept him from leaving the house and then convinced him to go to therapy. The crisis of his marriage and the abandonment of his wife, who left him alone with their two children, had worn him out considerably. Aldo was very rigid, he had an obsessive personality with depressive traits, and joins the group in a moment of profound sadness because all his certainties about his family's stability have gone up in smoke. In group, surprisingly, he trusts others a lot, discusses openly with them, and thanks to their support, manages to face the separation from his wife and take responsibility for the custody of their children in a healthy, non-destructive way. The awareness of having been a house of stone and a bear will lead him to open up and reveal his emotional richness to the group: It is in the dream space that he finds himself ready to start a new affective life.

Conclusions

Dreams are a powerful language evocative of profound script scenarios and the change that accompanies therapy. Listening to the language of an adult's dreams means gaining access to the level of the Child ego state with greater immediacy, as a child therapist does with drawings and games. The group functions as an imposing theatrical stimulus and a receptacle for emotions, suggestions, and images, similar to that of the mother described by Bion (1992) in the processes of reverie. In this way, the group gives rise to the oneiric climate that nurtures the reactivation of the Child dreamer who has written the script and who can rewrite it according to a new plan within a matrix of new decisions, new perspectives, and new options.

Furthermore, dreams provide a way to access themes that are not accessible at the verbal and conscious level of memory and thought, especially in traumatized clients, as Moccia (2012) writes, commenting on Schore and Bucci's work:

> There is no possible narration when the traumatic experience has been inscribed into memory before the advent of the symbolic skills, and, since the mind never really gives up the search for meaning and affective communication, these contents find a first expression in the acted-on, the transference repetitions and the projective identification, and a first iconic-symbolic articulation in dreams.
>
> (Bucci, 1997; Moccia, 2012)

A client, Licia, one night toward the end of her group treatment, brings up a very meaningful dream:

> *I'm with one of my high school friends and we both come to you (the therapist). He was my lover at the time and he comes up to you and you welcome him into your arms and I see how he surrenders himself to you, enjoying this hug in a way I couldn't have done. In the dream, I was looking at him with tenderness and a good kind of envy, and I think I'd like to be able to let myself go during hugs, too.*

In the analysis of the dream, Licia points out how she is very happy of the dream's emotional trail: "I wasn't envious as I was all my life, my envy was the desire to surrender myself to affection."

The group tells Licia that she has changed very much, that she is now capable of this surrender, that she has transformed her hostility and envy and that that is apparent to everyone.

The exchange terminates with everyone being deeply moved, even though the session is taking place online in this time of Covid.

Note

1   Mentalization is the ability to "think" one's own mental states as well as others' (feelings, desires, intentions, and thoughts themselves); it lies at the heart of human beings' capacity to be in relation with each other, that is, to be a "social animal," as Aristotle used to say (Fonagy, 2001).

References

Berne, E. (1957). *A layman's guide to psychiatry and psychoanalysis*. New York: Simon & Schuster.

Berne, E. (1966). *Principles of group treatment*. Oxford: Oxford University Press.

Berne, E. (1972). *What do you say after you say hello? The psychology of human destiny*. New York: Bantam Books.

Bion, W. (1992). *Cogitations*. London: Karnac Books.

Bowater, M. (2001). The Fern monster: A one-session cure with dreamwork. *Transactional Analysis Journal, 31*, 258–261. doi:10.1177/036215370103100408

Bowater, M. (2003). Windows on your inner self: Dreamwork with transactional analysis. *Transactional Analysis Journal, 33*, 37–44. doi:10.1177/036215370303300106

Bowater, M. (2008). Facing the fear of death. *Transactional Analysis Journal, 38*, 151–154. doi:10.1177/036215370803800208

Bowater, M. (2009). Shutting out the dog: The value of nightmares in recovering from sexual abuse. *Transactional Analysis Journal, 39*, 149–152. doi:10.1177/036215370 903900208

Bowater, M. (2010). Redeeming the fruit fly: Redecision work with a recurring dream. *Transactional Analysis Journal, 40*, 95–98. doi:10.1177/036215371004000203

Bowater, M. (2013). Fighting back: Addressing a nightmare in counseling. *Transactional Analysis Journal, 43*, 38–47. doi:10.1177/0362153713486108

Bowater, M., & Sherrard, E. (1999). Dreamwork treatment of nightmares using transactional analysis. *Transactional Analysis Journal, 29*, 283–291. doi:10.1177 %2F036215379902900408

Bowater, M., & Sherrard, E. (2011). Ethical issues for transactional analysis practitioners doing dreamwork. *Transactional Analysis Journal, 41*, 179–185. doi:10.1177/036215371104100215

Bucci, W. (1993). The development of emotional meaning in free association. In J. Gedo & A. Wilson (Eds.), *Hierarchical conceptions in psychoanalysis* (pp. 3–47). New York: Guilford.

Bucci, W. (1997). Symptoms and symbols: A multiple code theory of somatization. *Psychoanalytic Inquiry, 17*(2), 151–172. doi:10.1080/07351699709534117

Bucci, W., Severino, S. K., & Creelman, M. L. (1991). The effects of menstrual cycle hormones on dreams. *Dreaming, 1*, 263–275.

Clarkson, P. (1992). *Transactional analysis psychotherapy: An integrated approach*. London: Tavistock, Routledge.

Fonagy, P. (2001). *Attachment theory and psychoanalysis*. New York: Other Press.

Foulkes, S. H. (1964). *Therapeutic group analysis*. London: Allen & Unwin.

Jung, C. G., Franz, M. L., Henderson, J. L., Jaffé, A., & Jacobi, J. (1964). *Man and his symbols*. Garden City, NY: Doubleday.

Moccia, G. (2012). *Commento alla relazione di A. Schore "Un cambiamento di paradigma nell'approccio terapeutico agli enactments"*. Retrieved from www.spiweb.it/ricerca/ moccia-g-2012-commento-alla-relazione-di-a-schore-un-cambiamento-di-paradigma-nellapproccio-terapeutico-agli-enactments-roma-20-e-21-ottobre-2012/

Neri, C., Pines, M., & Friedman, R. (2002). *Dreams in group psychotherapy: Theory and technique*. London: Jessica Kingsley.

Novellino, M. (1998). *L'approccio clinico dell'analisi transazionale*. Milano: Franco Angeli.

Siegel, D. J. (1999). *The developing mind: How relationships and the brain interact to shape who we are*. New York: Guilford Press.

Summers, G., & Tudor, K. (2005). Co-creative transactional analysis. In W. F. Cornell, H. Hargaden, & J. R. Allen (Eds.), *From transactions to relations: The emergence of a relational tradition in transactional analysis*. Chadlington, Oxfordshire: Haddon Press.

Winnicott, D. W. (1971). *Playing and reality*. London: Penguin.

15

EFFICACY OF TA PSYCHOTHERAPY GROUPS IN THE TREATMENT OF PERSONALITY DISORDERS

By now, the field of research on group psychotherapy is scientifically solid, and has produced, in the last 20 years, important results regarding the clinical efficacy of such a treatment (Burlingame, MacKenzie, & Strauss, 2004).

Several studies have underlined specifically how long-term psychodynamic group therapies (Lorentzen, Sexton, & Høglend, 2004; Sigrell, 1992; Tschuschke & Anbeh, 2000) are effective in the treatment of clients suffering from serious mental disorders, such as substance abuse and personality disorders, as well as in the treatment of victims of sexual abuse.

Since a personality disorder is a severe pathological condition involving different but interrelated functioning areas – the self, family, and parental relationships, social or group relationships – it also requires particularly incisive models of treatment able to directly influence not only the area of the self but also the more specifically relational one.

The ability to mentalize – to recognize that others have a different mind than our own –, which represents a psychological breakthrough for the individual, is considerably inhibited in these subjects, especially when it comes to attachment relationships (Bateman & Fonagy, 2006). Their P_1 is split, and, consequently, others are perceived as either good objects – Rescuers guaranteeing security and protection – when clients project their P_{1+} on them; or bad objects – powerful and destructive Persecutors – when they project their P_{1-} (Vignozzi, 2014). The boundaries of the self come off as fuzzy and this prevents these clients from experiencing both group members and therapist as individuals separate from themselves. The lack of boundaries between self and others corresponds to the mechanism of identity diffusion regarded by Kernberg (1975) as a one of the main traits of clients suffering from personality disorders. Such clients are not in touch with themselves, lack an integrating Adult, and are incapable of describing themselves to a significant other. This is a mechanism which contributes to twist interpersonal interactions, chronically disturbing them and generating an absence of reflective thinking and emotional regulation. In group therapy, identity diffusion happens above all when clients with personality disorders are involved in somebody else's problems: they get lost in them, entering an anxious state and confusing their own mind with the other's, they distance themselves from others

DOI: 10.4324/9781003215547-16

and become withdrawn, or they get too involved manifesting violent conflict. The twisted perception of themselves and others engenders unstable behaviors: clients might become either histrionic or inhibited, either passively withdrawn or aggressive, either grandiose or humble, either persecutors or masochists. When in the therapy group they realize that they share several traits with those they initially thought unacceptable, their hostile behavior softens and they slowly begin to integrate their own internal split and primitive representations.

For such clients, the authentic exchanges of the therapy group often comprise the only moments in which they receive feedback on the effects their personality model have on others, facilitating a decontamination process and the development of a secondarily adjusted group imago, where all members can see themselves for who they really are. Clients with personality disorders present a challenge for group psychotherapists because of the intensity of the affective responses they provoke in others.

They possess the ability to generate anger, disappointment, frustration and feelings of inadequacy. In particular, subjects with borderline and narcissistic personality disorders facing serious deficits of mentalization, as we shall see in the relevant paragraphs, tend to render communication more "acted-out" than "verbalized." On the other hand, it is also true that, if the group is heterogeneous, members possessing an integrated Adult will support the therapist in diluting the countertransference, increasing the therapist's reflective thinking. Since the latter is not directly involved in the moments of interaction between members, the therapist acts as an auxiliary "third eye" and manages to better stimulate the metacognitive function. At the same time, each member, when not directly engaged, has the possibility to observe the different interactions between fellow members, as well as between these and the therapist, carving out a time and space of reflection that is often impossible to find in individual therapy, as we observed in the chapter on transference and countertransference. In group, clients suffering from personality disorders experience strong emotions such as fear, anger, and sense of exclusion. Old traumas are enacted once again, with the same old patterns of behavior, but the therapist's calm approach offers the mirroring that is needed to cooperatively assign meaning to the symptom, the malaise. The pretensions of the client's self are thus put into perspective and, at the same time, the client's innate need to feel part of a narrative bigger than them is finally satisfied.

Thus, group therapy represents an extremely fertile context for the elaboration of interpersonal dynamics within a safe space, which favors reflective processes and discourages acting out.

Clients with borderline personality disorder

According to some authors, a combination of group and individual therapy – with the same therapist – is recommended in the treatment of clients suffering from borderline personality disorder. That is due to the propensity of such clients to activate defense mechanisms related to splitting (Rutan, Stone, & Shay, 2014).

These clients are rather intolerant when it comes to individual treatment because of the intense intimacy created by this dual dimension. The invalidating problems due to transference and countertransference emerge with extreme intensity. The absurd requests and the primeval anger – an anger that clients often act out through lateness, absences, and use of substances before a session – make individual treatment particularly draining for the therapist. Rutan and Alonso (1982) argue that the dropout percentage in group is significantly reduced when clients are also attending individual sessions.

Despite evidence proving the efficacy of group therapy for borderline personalities, these clients' primitive emotions and twisted perception of themselves and others participate in the creation of a perfect breeding ground for the therapist to lose control of the thought-processing dynamics. Group psychotherapy may also engender psychic withdrawal and a resort to action instead of verbalization, the exact opposite of what should be its goal. Another option is that in group, clients may exhibit dominant or openly controlling behaviors, openly rejecting the other's help and putting themselves at the center of everyone's attention, so as to satisfy their exhibitionistic needs. The hostility they provoke feels rather familiar to them and protects them from the danger of intimacy. They tend to continuously activate dramatic relationship schemes that see the therapist and fellow members in the role of Rescuer/Persecutor and themselves in the role of Victim/Persecutor.

During the activation of the Drama Triangle (Karpman, 1968) all script beliefs are made explicit and the client fluctuates between feeling helpless (V) and perceiving others as culpable for not being able to help them (P). The use of the Drama Triangle may have an educational function, encouraging borderline clients to consider the ways they participate in the success, or more often, the failure of their relationships. With this type of clients it is recommended to avoid extended silences, since that may trigger their fear of abandonment.

Because of their inability to recognize the effect they have on others, borderline clients react with surprise, pain, and, sometimes, anger to feedback from fellow group members; in such cases, it is important that the therapist empathize with their surprise instead of pushing them to accept the feedback. Legitimizing their difficulties is useful in order to strengthen security in the group climate, as well as to offer a space of reflection related to their lack of understanding of emotional cues or of other's intentions (Rutan et al., 2014). Additionally, with this strategy it is possible to avoid the risk for the borderline client to become a scapegoat, Victim of a group which becomes their Persecutor. For example, to a client angry about being confronted by another member on the hyper-detailed, boring way she recounts the events of her life, it would be useful to say:

> I understand you feel hurt because of what was said to you, but you have received this particular criticism also outside the group, as you said many times before, and here you have the possibility to understand your behaviors and transform them. Do not forget that this is the reason you

are here, to learn to accept other people's points of view, even if we are all aware of how difficult that is for you.

It is also necessary to stop a borderline client from pouring excessive anger on their fellow members without explaining their reasons, instead inviting the client to reflect on what they hope to achieve by expressing this anger: Is it being considered an "aggressor" by fellow members and risking isolation, or is it trying to reflect together with the whole group on the meaning behind this emotion, validating their need to be understood?

Clearly, the therapist's interruption does not always lead to borderline clients redefining themselves appropriately, but allowing anger to explode without containment may lead to them becoming a scapegoat, someone to avoid, to keep at arm's length. With a more mature client, it would be more helpful to explore their maladaptive models using interpretation techniques; instead, with borderline clients that would mean risking to feed into their anger and frustration, while supportive techniques have proven more effective.

The purpose of keeping to the here-and-now and resorting to the client's past only to understand how their script is influencing their present is to energize and integrate their Adult, who learns to recognize the subjective difference between their own mental states and those that are being offered to them by fellow members.

Another useful technique consists in underlining the similarities shared by other members with respect to the client's concerns and defense style. This approach tends to keep peer transactions fluid. As it happens, because of their emotional intensity, such clients often challenge and threaten fellow members, forcing them to face the similarities they share with others.

Oscar, the client we met in Chapter 5, used to often look impatiently at the clock every time. Simone, a very shy group member, talked haphazardly about his problems with his partner, stumbling through his words, often interrupting himself, and looking deeply embarrassed. During a session, a fellow group member pointed out to Oscar that his reaction was disrespectful and irritating; faced with this negative feedback, Oscar defended himself arguing that nobody could ever say they enjoyed or appreciated Simone's perspective, since it was always so difficult to follow. Some members openly declared that they also found Simone boring, but this boredom was bearable because the underlying theme, relationship trouble, involved everyone, and, after having explained everything, Simone always actively interacted with the others, chasing the boredom away. The therapist's remarks on boredom as a shared element and, most of all, on the fact that Simone's fear of resulting boring to others prevented Simone from being spontaneous and smooth in his narrative of self, managed to placate Oscar's anger, keeping him from becoming a container for the other's undesirable aspects and allowing him to adopt a different, more accepting behavior toward Simone. Oscar understood that he was voicing a shared emotion and, because he was legitimized instead of judged, despite the aggressive way in which he expressed his feelings, he was able to process and transform said emotion in a coherent thought, and thus to alter it. After this group session, his behavior toward Simone became less aggressive, he stopped looking at the clock and started to help him out of his embarrassment, while his aggression shifted toward other, less fragile, members, who were better at defending themselves.

Dissociation is that primitive defense mechanism that borderline clients resort to more easily when faced with affective states of excessive intensity. Traumatic relationships become inner parts whose function is to express a Victim/Persecutor dynamic, Parent/Child ego state relational units, that are projected onto fellow members, the therapist or their own person.

The mind of a client suffering from such a disorder might be compared to a group, which is a metaphor dear to transactional analysts. The individual mind possesses a collective dimension, a sort of stage, hosting different companies and plays. Actors are our ego states, telling stories and acting, in a healthy individual, with coherence and awareness, in harmony with other actors, all led by a director, the Adult. In the inner world of borderline personalities, each actor acts on their own: many dissonant voices, rigid roles, tragic caricatures of a Persecutor self, and a Victim self. The past prevails: negative feedback from a fellow member might take the client back to the voice of a stern mother, the therapist's remarks are experienced as abandoning and accepting them proves almost impossible, since they carry the silence of a distant father.

Rosenfeld compared the mind of a client with narcissist or borderline personality disorder with a mob gang:

> [It is] As if one were dealing with a powerful gang dominated by a leader, who controls all the members of the gang to see that they support one another in making the criminal destructive work more effective and powerful. . . . To change, to receive help, implies weakness and is experienced as wrong or as failure.
>
> (Rosenfeld, 1987, pp. 111–112)

Rosenfeld's words describe an inner world peopled by a group of characters overpowering the individual who hosts them and preventing them from integrating all their loving, constructive, and ethical parts.

By repeatedly acting out in the course of group therapy, we encounter those fragile aspects of personality that borderline clients cannot bear and "must" project at all costs on others, dissociating these from themselves. More than others, shame and humiliation are unbearable and impossible to contain within the inner world of such a client, who is subjugated by a critical "boss/Parent" controlling access to vulnerable emotions.

Nicola and Mary's case

Nicola, a client suffering from borderline personality disorder who has been in the group for a year now, speaks disdainfully to Mary – whom we have encountered before in the chapter on therapeutic alliance (Chapter 7) and who was expressing the trouble she has interacting with her teenage son. He points out to her that while she was "yammering on" she made a grammar mistake using a tense instead of another. "You can't even speak proper Italian, shame on you! No wonder your son feels superior to you! Learn how to speak before you open that mouth!" A deadly silence falls upon the room. Mary is frozen in place, her cheeks burning with shame, her eyes staring into nothingness, her shoulders bending forward, as if she was a piece of clothing from under which someone just took away the hanger. The therapist, perceiving a deep anger toward Nicola and his arrogant and violent words, turns to Mary trying to meet her eyes, but she is unable to establish direct eye contact with anyone. Beatrice, a member who is very close to Mary, tries to defend her, making a joke about the mistake in order to minimize the situation and bring some levity back into the room, but in vain. In the past, Mary often spoke about the many humiliations suffered at school due to her mother's psychosis, in the little southern town where she grew up. She was often a victim of bullying, and in the here-and-now of the group she has become once again that same tormented Child, petrified by shame, guilty of being the daughter of a weird mother who had to be hidden from the rest of the world. The therapist takes her time before intervening, deciding to keep silent, aware of the fact that her anger toward Nicola can be dangerous and runs the risk of heightening the client's aggressive enactments. She also knows that she can dampen his hostility by focusing on Nicola's Child, who was also a victim of bullying in his childhood and whose father used to be violent toward his mother. When a client manifests his hostility in such an intense manner, the rest of the group is often unable to say anything, as if they lacked the courage to intervene and, in their terror, preferred to express some sort of passive disengagement. They all look at Mary and the therapist, perhaps wishing for one of them to utter a magic word in order to ease the heavy tension looming over the group. Nicola is still, arms folded and legs outstretched, his gaze is fixed on Mary as well, as if he were proud of having humiliated her. "Mary, what's happening? What are you feeling right now": the therapist's voice is soft and sweet, her body leaning forward in order to show her closeness to her. She tries to syntonize with Mary's shame through her face's proxsemic cues, right brain to right brain. Mary starts to cry and slowly begins to describe the humiliation and fatigue she felt when, as a teenager, she moved to Tuscany from the south and her nightmare was not being able to speak proper Italian and falling back into her southern dialect. She had forgotten about this detail related to language, having dissociated it from her mind. She tells the group how she was tormented by her classmates because she was different, because her mother was known as "the crazy lady." The group supports and comforts her in her grief: Others have been bullied in the past and it is not difficult to participate in Mary's pain and share it. It is the first time Mary's account is truly authentic and integrated with past emotional experiences, and thanks to the intensity of her narration we can touch the splinters of her suffering and maybe even others', Nicola's included, who shifted on his chair so as to lean toward Mary as well. Mary's previous narrations had been lacking emotion. She seemed to regard herself as someone unworthy of other people's attention, just a thing that needed to be fixed. "What should I do?" was what she usually said after she had finished describing her issues, as if she was only there to figure out the best way to be accepted, as if her head did not work and she had to avoid showing her "insanity" to others. Dissociating to escape oneself and one's own subjectivity, especially as a reaction to shame: this is the mechanism shared by Nicola and Mary, a withdrawal in the Child/Parent relational state units which prevent the Adult from building an organic narrative. Nicola's anger was instrumental in order to dredge up long-forgotten fragments of Mary's history and reexperience them in the presence of "benevolent witnesses" willing to let themselves be transported into her past (Ferenczi, 1988/1932).

When a more relaxed and intimate atmosphere has been reestablished in the group, the therapist turns to Nicola, whose face now expresses pain and guilt, but the session is coming to an end and the therapist worries he is going to skip the following one, as it happened already sometimes in the past:

> I might be wrong but I think you understand what Mary is feeling right now because you have also felt it in the past. When you're ready to talk about what happened tonight, you will, because I believe it might be important for you, Mary and the group to understand what brought about that violent burst of anger. I only ask that you don't skip the next sessions, because it really is crucial

> for you to understand what lies behind your need to attack others. Your anger allowed Mary to contact something deep and authentic within herself and I'd like for it to do the same for you.
>
> Nicola will then attend the following sessions and talk about the sadness hidden behind his anger, as well as his regret to have hurt Mary in such a way.

Both Mary and Nicola suffer from personality disorders: Mary from dependent disorder, Nicola from borderline disorder. The latter often plays the role of the manipulator or Persecutor in the group, as we have just seen, but the fact that the group is composed of rather mature members, who have been in group longer than him, helps him contain his explosions of anger and, over the subsequent sessions, reflect on what led him to attack Mary in such an arrogant manner. What emerged was that Mary is the most fragile person, but also the one that Nicola felt closest to, and he is terrified of closeness. They both enacted in group what happens in their individual minds: a Persecutor who either torments and humiliates a helpless inner Victim or externalizes their attacks toward "Victims" in flesh and blood. Both Nicola and Mary suffer from eating disorders and they alternate between gaining and losing weight, which is apparent to everyone in group: their bodies are Victims of their internalized Persecutors. Mostly, Nicola tends to identify with the Persecutor, while Mary with the Victim, and this makes them very similar as well as very different, because we are most afraid and angry at the parts of the others we recognize in ourselves. Judith Butler argues:

> If my fate is not originally or finally separable from yours, then the "we" is traversed by a relationality that we cannot easily argue against; or, rather, we can argue against it, but we would be denying something fundamental about the social conditions of our very formation.
>
> (2004, pp. 22–23)

Clients with narcissistic personality disorder

The narcissistic personality disorder has always been object of intense discussion among clinicians and scholars because of its complex and multiform nature, so much so that it ran the risk of being erased from DSM-5 (American Psychiatric Association, 2013). The addition of the dimensional assessment of personality to the classic categorical one in section III of personality disorders in the aforementioned manual represented the final compromise that allowed the narcissistic disorder to be recognized and its interactive dimensions to be described.

161

When we discuss the disorder in question, we believe it is necessary to consider the differences between thick and thin-skinned narcissism, as indicated by Rosenfeld (1987), or overt and covert narcissism, according to Cooper (1988), or grandiose and vulnerable narcissism, according to Pincus and Roche (2011). We can trace back the description of the many subtypes of narcissisms to the gap between Kernberg's (1975) and Kohut's (1971) thoughts: the first attributes to the client suffering from narcissistic disorder a grandiose personality with exhibitionistic traits, while the second considers them fragile and hypersensitive.

However, these distinctions are rarely that pronounced in the clients we have encountered in the course of our practice. A client who appears to be grandiose and self-assured might break down following a rejection or the onset of old age, the same way that a hypersensitive and vulnerable client might manifest angry and scorned reactions if they feel narcissistically wounded. The problem shared by all clients suffering from this type of disorder is their poor perception of others (Gabbard, Miller, & Martinez, 2006), and that is why group therapy might prove extremely effective.

Inserting a client with narcissistic disorder in group, however, may reveal to be a rather complicated feat, because of all the aspects mentioned earlier. It is clearly useful for these subjects, since it puts them face to face with other members' needs and the subsequent impossibility to always be at the center of everyone's attention, but it may also become a double-edged sword. On the one hand, they like the idea of having a public at their disposal; on the other, they cannot bear to share their time with others or to receive negative feedback.

Although at a first glance they might appear rather integrated in social interactions and they generally have better impulse control than clients with borderline disorder, they actually lack empathy. In the previous paragraph, we have seen how Oscar, who suffer from borderline personality disorder, after having processed his aggression toward Simone, started to support and help the latter with the troubles he had narrating himself. Meanwhile, clients with narcissistic personality see themselves as special, feel like it is in their right to receive special attentions from the therapist, rarely ask any questions or show interest and support toward others. For such clients, too, it is recommended combining group therapy with individual therapy by the same therapist (Gabbard et al., 2006; Bateman & Fonagy, 2006) in order to deeply process their rejection of the other's perspective and the other themselves. Klein and Bernard (1994) suggest group treatment with co-conduction by two therapists, so as to be able to properly deal with the complex countertransference reactions elicited by clients with narcissistic disorder and manage the unstable trend of intense transference reactions. It is crucial that the two therapists have a years-long well-established work relationship, as well as be available to undergo supervised sessions so as to face possible countertransference dynamics.

At the root of many a transference reaction from a client with narcissistic personality we have, beside the split, the fluctuation between idealization and devaluation, strongly tied with the fluctuation between Parent and Child ego state. At times, these clients see the therapist as an almighty figure there to save them, while other times the therapist is seen as insensitive, cold and useless, someone to be destroyed. The group offers these clients the opportunity to correct such distortions and limit the extent of their fluctuations.

The most common game played in group is "Kick me": It is precisely because of this game that the dropout percentages of such clients are so consistent, since they often leave because they function as scapegoats. However, if they are persuaded to stay, we might be able to witness an important period of change. Devaluation and almighty control are the defense mechanisms these clients often employ in order to keep therapist and fellow members at arm's length: such mechanisms must be processed continuously in order for the treatment to be successful. One of the goals of therapy is to help these clients develop a sense of guilt and concern for others, which means structuring an inner Nurturing Parent that would help them empathize with their inner parts and with others.

A crucial step with them is interpreting the narcissistic wound, when it emerges, not as their individual wound but as belonging to the whole group, so as not to stigmatize them and build a shared understanding of the fact that their relationship styles represent efforts to sustain and protect their fragile parts. Another important task the therapist has to accomplish with these clients is to bring back their monologues to the here-and-now, in order for them to realize that there are other people with whom it is necessary to share time and attention.

Elena's case

Elena is about 40 years old. After two years of individual therapy, the therapist arranges for her to join a group, since their therapeutic work has slowed down and Elena is still keeping the people in her life at a distance, including the therapist. Elena is convinced her life will change only when she finds a handsome, rich, educated man with whom to start a family. She is a beautiful woman, was rather successful in her studies and works as researcher at a pharmaceutical company, where she is her boss' favorite. With the latter she has a friendly relationship, he is always advising her on how to keep the men she meets. The problem is that Elena's relationships with her partners are always short lived: the latter always feel pressured by her urge to change them so as to make them more what she needs them to be, thus after a while the pressure becomes overwhelming and they decide to leave.

At the fourth group session, Elena talks about the latest man she met on a dating site and that she started dating in the last month. He seems to possess all the qualities she desires: he is an engineer holding an important position at a famous tech company, he is handsome, funny, and apparently quite taken with her. Elena, however, is angry with him because he smokes

---

and at times drinks a beer too much when they go out. While they listen to her, the other three women in the group openly manifest their surprise and discomfort, opening their eyes wide and shifting nervously in their chairs. They then proceed to confront her on the fact that drinking two beers on a Saturday night is not the same as being an alcoholic, and that smoking is not an inappropriate behavior but simply a fragility some people have. They point out that the way she narrates herself is that of a Critical Parent who is always pointing the finger. One of them is a 50-year-old woman who has been separated for 20 years from a husband-child who refused to take care of their children, both economically and affectively. Another lives alone and suffers from eating disorders, is overweight and is too ashamed to date men. The third is a 35-year-old woman separating from a partner who in a way is similar to Elena, "she's only concerned about herself and her needs, exactly like you," she states. But their remarks fall short: Elena seems not to care at all. Even one of the men in the group, who is a smoker, tries to make her understand that such criticism toward a man she barely knows is exaggerated and she risks playing with him the "Now I've Got You, You Son of A Bitch" game. But Elena responds to everyone hurriedly starting all her sentences with "yes, but" the famous words of the game "Why Don't You – Yes, But" and continues to talk about what she deems most important: making her partner understand that if he wants to stay with her he has to stop smoking and drinking! Not only that, but she keeps listing all his shortcomings, such as loving a house with a garden, nature, and the sea, while she wants to live in the city. Hers is an endless monologue; she fails to realize the surprise and irritation she might elicit in fellow members, since they do not really exist: Elena is alone in the group as she is alone with the men she meets, lacking an Adult capable of reflecting on others' responses and, as a consequence, changing her way of thinking. The atmosphere within the group gets tenser by the minute. Only Mario, who also possesses some narcissistic traits and behaves in a similar way with his partner (in the previous session he told everyone how she had decided to leave him after discovering he had cheated on her once again), tries to understand Elena's frustration, arguing that hers is still a fairly new relationship and it will probably take time to learn to negotiate each other's needs. Elena lets him speak and seems to calm down, as if she might be able to accept being influenced by another only if the hope for change is presented to her in a way that overlooks her mistakes.

The therapist turns to Elena to ask her how she is feeling and what ego state is prevailing within her at the moment, since it feels like the work with her is going nowhere, same as her relationship with men. She also points out to Elena how her behaviors exclude the people around her, how the pressure she exerts on others causes everyone to leave her, the same way she feels alone when faced with a man she wants to change at all costs even before getting to know him and recognize him for what he really is: a person, with his limits and resources. Bringing back everything that happens outside to the here-and-now of the group allows everyone to open up to the reality of limits, one's own limits as well as others', and above all the limit of not having had perfect parents. To the therapist's request to explore her ego states Elena replies irritably: "I don't get it, you say I'm activating my Critical Parent, but I feel like a misunderstood Child!" "Obviously, for you it feels that way, but we cannot see that Child. Does it often happen to you that others see you differently than how you feel?" asks the therapist. Elena starts talking about her father and how he never really saw her, he always criticized her since in his eyes she was always "whining." She always felt like she lived in her brother's shadow, who, despite being much less diligent than her, was chosen by her father to lead the family's company. She recounts how her mother always treated her as a wunderkind, deserving of a man as perfect as her, who would make her happy for the rest of her life. Elena experiences for the first time, as she speaks, a sense of continuity of the self, and the group looks at her in a new way, recognizing the fragility and humanity of a person who is burdened by a past that made her similar to a steamroller, in her rush to prove to everyone her ability to maintain high performance standards. Toward the end of the session, Carla, a 50-year-old separated woman, asks tentatively: "Excuse my ignorance but, what's the magical world of Kinder?" and the entire group bursts out laughing! At the beginning, Elena told everyone she had met her current boyfriend "in the magical world of Tinder" and Carla's expression will become an inside joke for the group. Every time Elena, in subsequent sessions, will mention her boyfriend's shortcomings, with whom she is still in a relationship six months after the session herein described, there will always be a group member to remind her: "Remember that the magical world of Kinder doesn't exist! Come back to the real world!"

We do not know if Elena will ever be cured of her almightiness and her need to change others. What we do know is that group therapy forces her greedy and almighty Child to take responsibility of her limits: each individual's freedom stops where another's begins. Elena is finding herself in the mind of the group, and it happens every time she makes sense of her inability to see others: she was overlooked by her father or she was seen as a narcissistic object by her mother (Marconcini, 2020). Her Child's vulnerable parts are also emerging and she can better distinguish her own mental states as well as others'. Individual therapy, on its own, would have failed to help her reach this awareness in the course of just a few months. "It is very possible that one benefit of group therapy is that therapy in groups often promotes mentalization" (Widdowson, 2010, p. 332). It is clear that Elena's sense of responsibility is not set forever: at times, during her most difficult moments, she goes back to steamrolling, creating tensions among members. However, in these dialectic moments, she is accompanied by a shared group thought, a group Adult, able to contain and make sense of her need of almightiness that, at the same time, renders her helpless.

Conclusions

Personality disorders are to be considered as falling into a "wide middle ground" (Lingiardi, 2018): people suffering from them are neither neurotic nor psychotic, since they are less organized than neurotics but more integrated than psychotics. And defining a client with a personality disorder must not be considered a way to label and reify their human experience.

The diagnosis, according to PDM-2, must remain an open question for the clinician, because the clinician is not interested in the disorder itself but in the client suffering from that particular disorder. For this reason, the authors of PDM-2 prefer the expression "a taxonomy of people" over "a taxonomy of disorders" (Lingiardi & McWilliams, 2017, p. 2).

The diagnosis must remain an open question, especially when it comes to personality disorders, since it is a pathology with a great variety of clinical manifestations and comorbidity with other disorders requiring the clinician's attention and mental flexibility.

Classification systems and tests are not enough to diagnose personality disorders. The interview, on the contrary, is a much better context; the encounter with the client's subjectivity provides hypothesis for a therapeutic plan that is really adequate to the needs of the individual client without excluding the needs of remaining group members. In this chapter, we have tried to demonstrate the complexity of these disorders, which are often hard to treat through individual therapy.

Although the diagnosis will never be exact, we know that such personality structures are extremely vulnerable and may benefit significantly from group therapy, as we have seen, because the group allows the clients to conduct a powerful and accurate reality testing. In this textbook, the majority of clinical cases involve clients suffering from such disorders precisely because today, given their characteristics, these are considered among the most widespread and debilitating psychopathologies.

To be part of a therapy group means to belong to the interpersonal world and these clients in particular have a burning need to feel this sense of belonging. In group, they will not find joy or liberation from pain, but they will acquire the ability to perceive themselves as people among people, to make sense, with others, of pain and joy. In group, the stories revolving around them are shared by them in a space located half-way from who they are today and who they would like to be in the future.

References

American Psychiatric Association. (2013). *Diagnostic and statistical manual of mental disorders* (5th ed.). Arlington, VA: Author. doi:10.1176/appi.books.9780890425596

Bateman, A., & Fonagy, P. (2006). *Mentalization-based treatment for borderline personality disorder: A practical guide.* Oxford: Oxford University Press. doi:10.1093/med/9780198570905.001.0001

Burlingame, A., MacKenzie, K. R., & Strauss, B. (2004). Small group treatment: Evidence for effectiveness and mechanisms of change. *Handbook of Psychotherapy and Behavior Change, 5,* 647–696.

Butler, J. (2004). *Precarious life: The powers of mourning and violence.* London: Verso.

Cooper, A. M. (1988). The narcissistic-masochistic character. In R. A. Glick & D. I. Meyers (Eds.), *Masochism: Current psychoanalytic perspectives* (pp. 117–138). Hillsdale, NJ: Analytic Press, Inc.

Ferenczi, S. (1988). *The clinical diary of Sándor Ferenczi* (M. Balint & N. Z. Jackson, Trans.). Cambridge, MA: Harvard University Press (Originally published in 1932).

Gabbard, G., Miller, L., & Martinez, M. (2006). A neurobiological perspective on mentalizing and internal object relations in traumatized patients with borderline personality disorder. In J. G. Allen & P. Fonagy (Eds.), *Handbook of mentalization-based treatment* (pp. 123–140). New York: Wiley. doi:10.1002/9780470712986.ch5

Karpman, S. (1968). Fairy tales and script drama analysis. *Transactional Analysis Bulletin, 7*(26), 39–43.

Kernberg, O. (1975). *Borderline conditions and pathological narcissism.* New York: J. Aronson.

Klein, R. H., & Bernard, H. S. (1994). Utilizing co-therapy in group treatment of borderline and narcissistic patients. In V. L. Schermer & M. Pines (Eds.), *Ring of fire: Primitive affects and object relations in group psychotherapy* (pp. 198–240). London: Routledge.

Kohut, H. (1971). *The analysis of the self: A systematic approach to the psychoanalytic treatment of narcissistic personality disorders.* Chicago, IL: University of Chicago Press.

Lingiardi, V. (2018). *Diagnosi e destino.* Torino: Einaudi.

Lingiardi, V., & McWilliams, N. (Eds.). (2017). *Psychodynamic diagnostic manual: PDM-2* (2nd ed.). New York: The Guilford Press.

Lorentzen, S., Sexton, H. C., & Høglend, P. (2004). Therapeutic alliance, cohesion and outcome in a long-term analytic group: A preliminary study. *Nordic Journal of Psychiatry, 58*(1), 3340. doi:10.1080/08039480310000770

Marconcini, A. (2020). Il narcisista e l'assertivo-vulnerabile. *Percorsi di Analisi Transazionale, VII*(2), 27–60.

Pincus, A. L., & Roche, M. J. (2011). Narcissistic grandiosity and narcissistic vulnerability. In W. K. Campbell & J. D. Miller (Eds.), *Handbook of narcissism and narcissistic personality disorder* (pp. 31–40). Hoboken, NJ: John Wiley & Sons.

Rosenfeld, H. A. (1987). *Impasse and interpretation: Therapeutic and anti-therapeutic factors in the psychoanalytic treatment of psychotic, borderline, and neurotic patients.* London: Routledge.

Rutan, J. S., & Alonso, A. (1982). Group therapy, individual therapy, or both? *International Journal of Group Psychotherapy, 32*(3), 267–282. doi:10.1080/00207284.1982.11492053

Rutan, J. S., Stone, W. N., & Shay, J. (2014). *Psychodynamic group psychotherapy.* New York: The Guilford Press.

Sigrell, B. (1992). The long-term effects of group psychotherapy: A thirteen-year follow-up study. *Group Analysis*, *25*(3), 333–352. doi:10.1177/0533316492253012

Tschuschke, V., & Anbeh, T. (2000). Early treatment effects of long-term outpatient group therapies – first preliminary results. *Group Analysis*, *33*(3), 397–411. doi:10.1177/0533316400333008

Vignozzi, F. (2014). Tra il regno e l'esilio: Narcisismo e transfert in psicoterapia. *Percorsi di Analisi Transazionale*, *1*, 33–54.

Widdowson, M. (2010). *Transactional analysis: 100 key points and techniques*. London and New York: Routledge.

16

DEPRESSIVE AND BIPOLAR DISORDERS IN A GROUP SETTING

The group as setting of choice in the treatment of mood disorders

The group is without a doubt a supportive container which provides people suffering from depression with a useful way to structure time, a system of strokes, meaningful social interactions, and a space and time where to gain awareness of their repressed emotions. In group, it is indeed possible to uncover the anger hidden behind apathy, understand its energetic value, and learn how to direct its force in order escape inertia and face life. For a depressed person who tends not to recognize their emotions, the group might thus become a psycho-educational experience, but above all a privileged site of exploration and self-knowledge.

In therapy, we often encounter people suffering from bipolar disorder, a disorder that might express itself through a wide range of symptoms, from cyclothymia to full-blown psychosis. When the person in treatment manifests a high degree of mood imbalance, as therapists know that we have to necessarily work with a method that integrates the psychotherapeutic process with pharmacological treatment. In such cases, the first goal is to stabilize the client's mood through decontamination of their Adult ego state. As a matter of fact, people suffering from this particular disorder, when in dysphoric and manic states, often reject medication, and this means frequent interruptions of treatment, as well as the repetition of severe depressive episodes which follow these delusions of grandeur. If the crazy Child prevails, the client refuses to listen to anyone, distrusts everyone, and breaks all bonds and alliances, including the one with the therapist. The client also tends to withdraw from treatment and isolate themselves when what prevails is the guilt tied to their introjected punitive Parent.

As stated in the second edition of the *Psychodynamic Diagnostic Manual* (2017), "Individuals with mania may have feelings of being strained, fragmented, and restless, as well as feelings of utter elation and absolute well-being. Their rapid mood fluctuations are accompanied by equally rapid fluctuations in the experience of self." Among the cognitive patterns we may find "fantasies of invincibility and exceptional, unrecognized talent" and, among the relationship patterns, unpredictability as well as "chaotic, impulsive, and highly sexualized" aspects.

DOI: 10.4324/9781003215547-17

For such reasons

> the psychodynamic treatment of bipolar states is likely to be daunting. Therapists may have trouble keeping up with the (hypo-)manic phases and may be bewildered by rapid shifts between these phases and depressed ones. The resultant confusion may spiral into countertransferential hostility.
>
> (pp. 159–160)

The difficulties experienced while treating this type of clients led us to experiment with integrated treatments in which individual psychotherapy is supplemented by group therapy and pharmacological treatment. When the relation with the therapist becomes difficult, as it happens, the group proves to be a grounding force and an even safer place for such clients.

Transactional analysis and studies on bipolar disorder

In transactional analysis, after Berne, who described the ego state structure of people suffering from bipolar disorder in terms of contaminations and exclusions (Berne, 1961, 1966), and Gouldings, who illustrated the injunctions tied to depression (Goulding & Goulding, 1978, 1979), Loomis and Landsman's contributions (1980, 1981) were fundamental to understand bipolar disorder.

According to the aforementioned authors, having parents who expressed a competitive reference system were centered from the very beginning on doing (or not doing) things, and manifested a grandiose approach to thoughts, feelings, and actions, constitutes in many cases the basis for the development of the manic depressive structure.

The use of denial as primary defense renders people suffering from bipolar disorder reticent to talk about their personal history. Oftentimes, they enter treatment because they are depressed, they may admit to having suicidal thoughts, they lament a lack of energy, a disinterest toward their job and a general lack of motivation. Associated with this inability to do things is a feeling of anxiety which emerges in the client's Child in response to a lack of strokes. The distinctive linguistic traits of this type of clients include kinesthetic expressions such as "running all over the place," "being hyper," "flying," "falling," and "running madly," which are uttered with an air of grandeur, rapidly, almost feverishly.

At times, this frenetic way of speaking makes listening to these clients rather tiring. Doing things, for them, is of the utmost importance.

Some are very successful and have trouble only when their success is somehow hindered, while others seem more at ease with failure and do their best not to be successful.

Hypomania is another common symptom which could lead such clients to get in touch with a therapist. Those suffering from it are unpleasantly hyper, their ideas are grandiose and their energy is squandered and unfocused. Moreover, they

170

fail to eat, sleep well, and take care of themselves, and their level of unrest often upsets people around them.

According to Loomis and Landsman (1981), the treatment has to be administered by a non-competitive point of view. These clients consider in a rather polarized way the contents of the sessions. They need a therapist playing the role of a realistically Nurturing Parent. A large majority of clients suffering from manic-depressive pathologies acts on the imaginary assumption according to which one day they will receive the fantasied nourishment, often approaching therapy with this expectation. The treatment and the therapist, too, will be considered as a polarized experience, of an "all or nothing" kind. It is especially important for therapists to avoid the setting of these grandiose expectations, sending clients messages such as "I will take care of you in a healthy way." That is because an unsatisfied grandiose expectation may be used by the client to drop out of treatment.

The description of the stages of treatment given by Loomis and Landsman (1981, pp. 347–348) still seems quite relevant to this day.

1   Lower defenses

  • set basic contracts
  • deal with behavioral manifestations
  • achieve and maintain social control

2   Decontamination work

  • confront grandiosity and discounting
  • emphasize use of Adult for problem solving
  • transactional and game analysis

3   Exclusion work

  • deal with developmental and script issues
  • provide realistic Nurturing Parent
  • provide integration messages

4   Integration

  • facilitate decision to alter (rather than adapt) structure
  • facilitate decision to give up fantasied Nurturing Parent
  • teach increased awareness and control of energy cathexis

5   Resolutions

  • facilitate natural, realistic use of options for thinking, feeling, and doing.

In our opinion, the most important goal of the first stage is to achieve and maintain social control in order to manage the behavioral manifestations of these clients.

The second stage, which might take place at the same time as the first, is devoted to decontamination. Here, the therapist focuses on the ability of the client to activate the Adult ego state when it comes to problem solving. Thus, the client can learn how to slow down and, before acting, examine the meanings behind the stimuli they receive. When the therapist suggests that the client adopts a more relaxed pace, it is possible that they might lament a decline in their Child's spontaneity (the excitement created by the manic Child).

"Most problems have a solution" and "You are able to solve problems" are the messages therapists have to offer to such clients when they come face to face with their manic-depressive grandiosity. "Fears of never getting enough, always being depressed, driving people away, or not being able to stand it are common" in this type of clients (Loomis & Landsman, 1981, p. 349).

During the decontamination process, therapists need to pay special attention to family transactions and the games used in order to play along with the script. The bottom line of these clients' script is to end up alone and cease to exist. That is the end result of such a script, both for clients who tend to seek others out, as well as for those who reject them.

The third stage focuses on problems tied to early development and the script. These clients tend to deny such problems. So, when they decide to take them into account that they may have trouble maintaining a consistent level of energy. Thus, they may experience sudden fears, transient sleep disorders and trouble keeping their Adult energized. Since for many clients these symptoms are related to their grandiose personality structure, in order not to reinforce this structure and the archaic decisions associated with it, therapists will need to encourage them to solve in a healthy manner those aspects of the problem the clients had discounted up until that moment.

In treating issues tied to the depressive stage, deconfusion work may also be effective. All clients suffering from borderline personality disorder, despite the variety of their disorder's manifestations, have in common an element of depression in infancy (which might make its first appearance, in some cases, as early as in infants aged 0–3 months). All people with manic-depressive traits share similar characteristics tied to their early development. Some clients have been hyper-protected, others abused; others were expected to always win, others to always fail; but the key issue for everyone is related to their own existence. Clients with manic-depressive traits have built an elaborate internal structure of exclusions, each of which must be identified, processed, and integrated.

The fourth stage focuses on structure and integration. Here, clients have the chance to alter their structure instead of adapting it. At this point, usually, clients have acquired an awareness and assumed control of their new energy cathexis, which has increased, since they have abandoned the practice of denying thoughts, feelings, and behaviors as a strategy toward problem-solving. Their decision to give up their fantasied Nurturing Parent facilitates in these clients the integration process – since it allows them to moderate the tendency to adaptation typical of both aspects of their structure – and grants them better access to their Natural Child. Their own Parent can thus be perceived in its more realistic dimension, free from its strictly competitive aspects. Feelings experienced in the here-and-now

172

and parental beliefs may now go hand in hand, without the need to resort to an external competitive system of exclusion and denial. It is in this moment that our clients should report feeling an integrated sense of self.

The fifth stage is that of resolutions. By now, the person in treatment should be able to identify the difference between "normal" excitement and previous manic episodes, as well as the difference between sadness due to loss and previous gloomy and solitary depressive episodes.

Loomis and Landsman's clients report being able to make normal and realistic use of the options at their disposal to think, feel and act with an excitement and spontaneity that is fun to share with others. This way, they will continue to develop as self-sufficient, flexible and productive individuals.

Michele Novellino (1988) wrote that

in the manic-depressive experience there is a real experience of loss (usually the loss of a loved object) which causes a regression of personality to oral and anal stages, causing, as a consequence, a reactivation of an ambivalence toward the object as well as the self.[1]

(p. 202)

Kapur (1987), in turn, draws a connection between TA theory and Arieti's psychoanalytic theory, which is based on the theme of the "dominant other," sought also in the person of the therapist by the depressed client (Arieti, 1977, p. 864). Recently, in the model described in his manual on the treatment of depressive states, Widdowson (2015) deemed useful to implement brief individual treatment programs of a cognitive approach, focused on the decontamination process.

In our experience, group treatment offers the possibility of working toward integrating the split structure, and thus allows a deep deconfusion process which would otherwise be hard to implement in a psychodynamic individual setting.

The clients' entrance into the group might take place in stage two or three of treatment, as per the Loomis-Landsman's model, after having carefully considered whether to integrate the group sessions with individual ones during moments of imbalance, either manic or depressive, and after having identified the best way to altogether facilitate pharmacological compliance.

Sara's case: From ugly duckling to swan

Sara has had a very difficult life: she grew up in a fragile family, with a father who could not take care of himself, let alone his family, and a childish mother who dreamt all her life to be rescued by a lover who kept her "on the back burner." At the age of 20 years, she starts having an endless series of depressive episodes, drops out of university several times, stops working.

After starting therapy with a passive attitude, in order to pay for treatment, she finds a job. She subsequently starts a paid vocational training course as a nurse, which she will end up completing successfully and which will allow her to find a stable job. Having concluded this first experience of psychotherapy, composed of two years of individual sessions and one year of group treatment, she starts applying for positions all around Italy, but in her self-sufficiency, it becomes apparent she is suffering from bipolar disorder: Sara alternates periods of excitement and hyperactivity characterized by weight-loss as well as frenetic and chaotic behaviors, and periods of hopelessness and apathy. She starts taking medications and reaches some sort of emotional stability. However, she is still restless and in pain. At the same time, she has to take care of an array of health issues regarding her family members, which, one after the other, get sick from cancer: first her uncle, who brought her up, then her father and grandmother. She is committed and attentive in her care for them, but soon she finds herself alone with her mother and a boyfriend who cannot fulfill the great emptiness she feels.

She begins a new cycle of psychotherapy when, newly married, at the age of 32 years, she is diagnosed with cancer herself. In psychotherapy, she finds the support she needs to face the facts of her disease and treatment, as well as the resolution to fight for her life. After a few years of intense treatment, she enters remission, and because of that her life goes back to normal, albeit interspersed by follow-up visits. In this stage, the group's support is especially helpful to her in order to "learn how to live and feel good," to use her words. Sara's problem at this point is that she cannot enjoy her life, cannot go on vacation, manage her finances, plan for good things, enjoy friendships and love, or have a laugh. During this time, therapy is especially helpful to Sara, who – officially declared cancer-free by the doctors – experiences a regression of her bipolar disorder, interrupts the pharmacological treatment, in agreement with her psychiatrist, and starts living and enjoying the "normal" things she rarely got to experience in the past.

A focus on Sara's behavior in group during the first cycle of treatment

Shortly after she joined the group, Sara starts arriving late and making spectacular entrances, interrupting fellow members, both to "apologize" and to announce her mood. During a guided fantasy suggested by the therapist to stipulate her individual contract in group, Sara describes herself as a "rambling rose on a wall" in which the flowers are few, beautiful and bright red, but they are also neglected as "the ones my mother keeps on her balcony." During the guided fantasy, the therapist suggests she imagine a gardener who can take care of the roses and make some changes, and Sara pictures a "a nice, good-looking guy, a professional, skilled figure, like the therapist." However, when she is asked to change her location, two discordant scenarios emerge, defined by Sara as "my usual extremes":

- I imagined myself in a forest, like a rose garden living on its own without the need of anything else;
- I imagined myself in a sunny garden, well cared for because I am "the only big, beautiful rose bed."

In both scenarios, Sara appears as the only one present, and the gardener is compared not merely to the magical therapist, but also to a dreamy Price Charming (hopefully a rich doctor) who would marry her and take care of her needs.

Processing and interpreting this material allow Sara to reveal to the group these archaic aspects of her script and develop an awareness of the fact that, in therapy, it is better to work toward "restructuring" rather than "adapting" her personality.

Her resistance manifests with repeated lateness and absences. In one such occasion, after having missed the previous session, Sara joins the group last, interrupting a conversation between members with: "Hello! Fancy meeting you here" and then "You know, I didn't want to come tonight. I don't feel good and I don't like people seeing me like this." In moments like these, the therapist's interventions are confrontational, so as to point out to her reticence to relate to her fellow members as an equal, but also the fact that her entrance, instead of interrupting the group process, can become a chance to work on the material it offers.

Session number ten of the first cycle of treatment

SARA: Basically, I miss therapy.
THERAPIST: Individual therapy?
SARA: Yes, the individual one!
THERAPIST: Then you're mad at me!
SARA: Yes, I am. Deep down, I am. Rationally, I'm not, but deep down in my guts, I am. All these people are fucking annoying. Don't take it personally, folks! But it's just fucking annoying. If they all disappeared right now and it was just you and me I'd slap you and I'd be happy. You know?
THERAPIST: [Laughing] Yeah, yeah.

SARA: Maybe it's because I don't have the most flexible schedule anymore. I mean, I was always late anyway, all the time, with more or less good excuses. But yeah, I was always late anyway.

THERAPIST: So you're saying this is not a recent problem.

SARA: No, it's just that now I feel it more 'cause, before, it used to be "my turn" all the time, and when I was in a good place I used to be in and out in less than an hour and I was super happy, so even if I was late it was okay, 'cause it was still my hour and I used to leave in a good mood. So the idea to have to come on the same day at the same time every week. . . . Maybe that's the problem.

THERAPIST: Did you know that one of the most important features of manic-depressive personalities is to have a competitive reference structure, based on "either me or them"? Either I exist or others do, either I'm the princess and always come first, or others can treat me like a doormat and step on me all the time.

SARA: You're scaring me. . .

THERAPIST: I'm telling you this because the thing you noticed is this competitive, rather primitive side of your feelings (which I've always seen in you), according to which you're either the only one that matters, or you end up at the extreme end of the spectrum, being the "mother" who's always putting other people first in spite of herself.

SARA: But that is my mom.

THERAPIST: Yes, that is obviously a model of relation you learned from her. That's where it started. That's why in a different situation you have trouble adapting. But you're still here, and you wouldn't always have stayed. You got "pissed," you got "mad," you got depressed a little, you "played hooky" a couple of times, but you came back, you told us, you're here and you're in an even better place than before. You're still aggressive, but not in the same way: Your aggression is now overt. You didn't come in saying "sorry" and then pushing everyone's buttons. . .

SARA: Yes, I'm consciously being aggressive, in this discussion.

THERAPIST: OK! That's important because now you can process that aggression, and that's the reason why, as I'd anticipated and I'm now confirming, group therapy represents a moment of growth for you.

SARA: Yes, you told me, it's not just about me. . .

THERAPIST: . . . Or just about them. It's about you *and* them, and being able to make space for ourselves *and* others makes us feel good. It makes us feel. . . . It's about setting healthy boundaries with others and create space for ourselves, which is basically the work we do in group and what you're doing now, telling us this.

SARA: [Laughs] People might get offended.

THERAPIST: They might, and if they do, they can tell you to your face if you offended them or not. And this is real, it mirrors reality back to us. After all, if I get "mad" at someone because they're here, they can also get "mad" at me, right? And I believe you can also face their anger. This is another experience you can have here. Someone here wants to tell us if they're angry?

MEMBER A: (lets out a noise between a yell and a moan)

THERAPIST: You agree?

A: Well, yeah!

THERAPIST: OK, Sara, welcome to the next stage. At this point it's very important to invite fellow members to talk if they have anything to say to you or if they feel like they can see themselves in you, because I sense both things here. Emotional reactions to what you said, but also mirroring.

GROUP: [Silence.]

THERAPIST: Any reactions to Sara's words? Or anyone mirroring them?

B: What do you mean by mirroring?

THERAPIST: Sharing what she feels when she says: "I'm annoyed I had to stop individual sessions," "I'd like to interact only with you," and "I'd like for the others not to be here."

SARA: But it's not like I wanted that. . .

THERAPIST: Let's hear from them now. [Toward B.] Why did you ask that question?

B: [Laughs] Maybe I do share that feeling.

THERAPIST: What did you feel while listening to Sara?

B: Well, maybe I was glad I was not alone in that.

THERAPIST: You were kind of enjoying it, weren't you?

B: [Smiles] Well, yeah!

SARA: I've got something important to say, though: It made me feel good, coming here, even though this part of me was always there and I could feel it. But coming here seemed useful to me too. That unwillingness was emotional, it's not like I didn't want to come. I mean, if I didn't, I wouldn't be here, right? That time I came here and they gave me strokes, that was important, beautiful . . . but it wasn't strong enough. It was a new experience but it was still very far away from me. In that moment, it was a strong message and it took me by surprise, but then, because this work is all new to me, it still wasn't strong enough to compensate for your messages, I mean when I would come here and talk about my week, and you would tell me what you thought would be gratifying for me, you gave me very clear, sharp inputs, you know?

THERAPIST: See, Sara, you're saying something important right now.

SARA: Well, you kind of are a parental figure for me. But I still miss it.

THERAPIST: Yes, and you said you accepted and enjoyed the positive strokes received during that experience in group. Now you're working toward integration. First, you told us about the problems and troubles you had with the group, and now you're telling us the other side of the coin. See? You're now integrating the difficult, problematic, negative parts of a relationship with the positive ones. And at the same time you told us that the positive emotions, the positive message, was so new to you that you had trouble contacting it.

SARA: Yeah, well, it did disappear pretty quickly.

THERAPIST: But that's because you're used to difficult relationships. Short term, even if you seek strokes, you can never fully accept them for yourself.

SARA: Yeah, I can never resist having a little dig at my boyfriend either.

THERAPIST: See, after all, you do feel comfortable in a state of conflict, in fights.

SARA: [Laughs.]

THERAPIST: Don't you?

SARA: Yeah, I do.

THERAPIST: Here, too, we can see some new, dissonant aspects, with respect to your past.

SARA: Well, yeah, when I'm here I try to avoid thinking just about my stuff and make an effort to listen instead, like, I try to avoid hiding in my problems and withdrawing from the world. I try to be here, for the others too, because it's good for me and them. Being together in an unconstructive way hurts all of us, hurts the whole group, and me and the others, all at the same time. And that's important because it puts everything in perspective, for me.

For example, her experience (A's) with anti-depressant, or hers (B's), we talked about it once, not in a session but outside, just the two of us: These are experiences that help me put things into perspective and make me feel that I'm not alone, that I can do it, that I need to push forward. Actually, when I get too much inside my head, I feel like I'm "fucking annoyed," like, I'm depressed and others are too: So fucking boring! That's a part of me I'm listening to now. But there's a different one: I really enjoyed talking to her (A), joining the group, talking to both you (A) and her (C).

But I always tell myself: I'm either unique or I'm nobody. So my depression is like: What others, I don't care about the others.

THERAPIST: You also told her. . .

178

SARA: Yes, I also told her she annoys the fuck out of me and [laughs]. . . .
I never went back to talk to that priest because he was confusing faith
with my feeling depressed. I wanna feel good even by myself, without
taking on more burdens like sin and guilt. . .

THERAPIST: Now that you said this, do you realize you refused to listen to
what she (A) was trying to tell you?

SARA: [Talking to A] What did you say?

A.: That I was pissed at you when you said you were the one who was suffering the most. I'm also suffering. And she was saying she was suffering
more than me. How do you know that? I don't see this as a competition.

SARA: I said that because. . .

THERAPIST: Stop. Feel what you're feeling right now. . . . What is it?

SARA: My defenses. . .

THERAPIST: Sara? What did you feel?

SARA: I don't know. I felt like I was seeing things from a different perspective, like I was present in the world with the others.

THERAPIST: So, it was a bit unpleasant, but you felt more in touch with
others.

SARA: Yes, I felt more normal, more normalized. Like something in me
was normal.

THERAPIST: And how did that make you feel?

SARA: Calm.

The exchange transcribed above took place while Sara was completing
her first therapy cycle. During this period she was active and present in the
group. She was working as a nurse in a hospital's surgical floor and at the
same time applying to become a psychiatric nurse. In a session before summer break, she said: "This group made me grow and now I'm sorry to be
separated from it."

Final observations on Sara's case

Sara's central themes emerged clearly during the first therapy cycle.
Observing the evolution of her life after the first cycle of therapy, we noticed
how her split defenses would kick in when she had to face commitments or
difficult moments like the illness and loss of her family members. Sara had
previously learned to take her medication regularly, how to ask for help and
go back to therapy in her most troubled moments. While she was sick with
cancer, she was strong and resolute, and she often said it was easier for her
to overcome cancer than depression. She discovered the pleasure of living
and her desire to invest in the future grew.

When, after five years of treatment and follow-up appointments, she is finally declared cancer-free, Sara gives birth to a little girl and proceeds to introduce her to the group and the therapist. She goes back to working as a nurse and asks for a health check in order to have her recovery formally recognized and the certification of disability for her bipolar disorder and oncological disease – which granted her facilitations on the job – officially revoked. "I feel good and I can work like anyone else," she declared with a certain amount of satisfaction.

Note

1   My translation.

References

Arieti, S. (1977). Psychotherapy of severe depression. *American Journal of Psychiatry*, *134*(8), 864–868. doi:10.1176/ajp.134.8.864

Berne, E. (1961). *Transactional analysis in psychotherapy: A systematic individual and social psychiatry*. New York: Grove Press.

Berne, E. (1966). *Principles of group treatment*. Oxford: Oxford University Press.

Goulding, M. M., & Goulding, R. L. (1978). Redecision: Some examples. *Transactional Analysis Journal*, *8*(2), 132–135. doi:10.1177/036215377800800208

Goulding, M. M., & Goulding, R. L. (1979). *Changing lives through redecision therapy*. New York: Grove Press.

Kapur, R. (1987). Depression: An integration of TA and psychodynamic concepts. *Transactional Analysis Journal*, *17*(2), 29–34. doi:10.1177/036215378701700206

Lingiardi, V., & McWilliams, N. (Eds.). (2017). *Psychodynamic diagnostic manual: PDM-2* (2nd ed.). New York: The Guilford Press.

Loomis, M. E., & Landsman, S. G. (1980). Manic-depressive structure: Assessment and development. *Transactional Analysis Journal*, *10*(4), 284–290. doi:10.1177/036215378001000403

Loomis, M. E., & Landsman, S. G. (1981). Manic-depressive structure: Treatment strategies. *Transactional Analysis Journal*, *11*(4), 346–351. doi:10.1177/036215378101100419

Novellino, M. (1988). *L'approccio clinico dell'analisi transazionale*. Milano: Franco Angeli.

Widdowson, M. (2015). Transactional analysis for depression: A step-by-step treatment manual. London: Routledge. doi:10.4324/9781315746630

17

THE END OF THERAPY

What does "end" mean?

The end of treatment in group therapy is usually a party, a celebration of the results achieved with respect to the initial contract, as well as a general improvement of health and quality of life.

The groups we have described up until now are semi-open groups in which a new client joins when another leaves, so as to keep the same number of members. Thus, each member reaches the end of group therapy when they have fulfilled their goals. It is usually up to the client to declare they want to put an end to their treatment and define a time for closure, which includes at least three sessions to process this ending and say goodbye to the group. In the course of their treatment, then, each member experiences the end of their fellow members' journeys and witnesses new people joining the group. The moments a new member joins or leaves are among the most important in each client's emotional experience and usually turn out to be the most indelibly imprinted in everyone's memory.

There is a time in the beginning in which clients join the group and introduce themselves to others. Subsequently, this self-introduction is repeated each time a new member enters the group. Members always refer to this as an important exercise that encourages them to be aware of their changes. So, when the time comes to separate themselves from the group and end their treatment, the self-introduction has changed considerably: it is usually richer and more open to the future.

Let's go back to the start

In the first stage of therapy, it is often suggested members do an exercise in which they are required to visualize and describe how they imagine themselves at the end of therapy, in order to help them develop a positive image of themselves. In some cases, therapists also suggest guided fantasies or group drawing techniques, so as to facilitate a representation of the self in the present moment and in the desired or feared future.

When, in the script questionnaires, the client is asked "Where do you imagine yourself in five years" or "at the end of your life," they are being encouraged

    DOI: 10.4324/9781003215547-18

to understand how the idea we have of us might influence our future, and take responsibility of the life they are building for themselves.

We have already mentioned how in the first stage we can observe the emergence of the clients' existential position, meaning, through the group imago, the idea they have of themselves, others and life. In terms of transference, we might say that what comes to the surface is the clients' Core Conflictual Relationship Theme (Luborsky & Crits-Christoph, 1990).

In some therapy group, we have videotaped each client's self-introduction and we have suggested they watch it at the end of their treatment, after having recorded a new one. The comparison between the two self-introductions is surprising and allows each member to crystallize their change. The same thing happens when we repeat the RAP interviews (Relationship Anecdotes Paradigm) at the end of therapy.

Some group therapists keep the text of the initial contract and suggest that members, in the final stage, re-read it together with the group in order to push them toward a self-evaluation of their own journey.

Sara's guided fantasy

We have already met Sara and her story in the chapter on depressive disorders.

As we have seen, shortly after joining the group, Sara starts arriving late and making rather dramatic entrances, interrupting others both to "apologize" and to announce her moods. During a guided fantasy suggested by the therapist to stipulate her individual contract in group, Sara describes herself as a "rambling rose on a wall" in which the flowers are few, beautiful and bright red, but they are also neglected as "the ones my mother keeps on her balcony." During the guided fantasy, the therapist suggests she imagine a gardener who can take care of the roses and make some changes, and Sara pictures a "a nice, good-looking guy, a professional, skilled figure, like the therapist." However, when she is asked to change her location, two discordant scenarios emerge, defined by Sara as "my usual extremes":

1 I imagined myself in a forest, like a rose garden living on its own without the need of anything else.
2 I imagined myself in a sunny garden, well-cared for because I am "the only big, beautiful rose bed."

In both scenarios, Sara appears as the only one present, and the gardener is compared not merely to the magical therapist, but also to a dreamy Price Charming (hopefully a rich doctor) who would marry her and take care of her needs.

Processing and interpreting this material allow Sara to reveal to the group these archaic aspects of her script and become aware that, in therapy, it is possible to work toward "restructuring" rather than "adapting" her personality.

The group as the third in the relationship

Jessica Benjamin (2017), a contemporary relationship psychoanalyst introduced us to the concept of the "Third" to define the space of the relationship and objectify it beyond duality. In our reading, Thirdness becomes the group, and it is through the group that clients can open themselves to Thirdness. It is akin to moving, in the Pythagorean Tetractys, from the number two, represented by a line, to the number three, represented by the triangle, which delineates a more complete space. Benjamin argues that in order to build this Thirdness it is necessary to "surrender to the Third," entering the dimension that Keith Tudor calls We-ness, the shared we in which the other's reality prevails on our mental pictures – the perceptions we have of others as represented by our mind.

In this process, which in transactional analysis is called the integrating Adult and the co-creative process, the client gives up the idealization of the Other, experiences the ambivalence of our own feelings as well as others', and accepts mistakes and the possibility of reparation.

They stop seeking perfection, preferring, instead, to look for a taste of real encounters with others and ourselves. When the experience of the group leads to a differentiation of the group imago, then it also inevitably leads to this maturation, this plunge into the real world.

Benjamin's concept of the Third also helps us move beyond the Freudian Oedipal model. According to the author, if we assume that a child, in order to grow and develop their identity, needs to have a mother and a father to encounter sexual difference, we risk promoting the idea that the acquisition/construction of identity evolves through an even, lineal process, thus denying, among other things, the very psychoanalytic notions of "fantasy," "sexuality," and "unconscious." We must consider the fact that this separation between active masculine and passive feminine constitutes none other than a reflection of our culture. What children truly desire is to identify with both parents in order to assimilate as many of their elements as possible. This model does not eliminate gender identity but allows each individual to express it with more flexibility and creativity, accepting all parts of ourselves and others, beyond social conventions. Thus, the Third becomes our capacity to observe ourselves from the outside, to integrate all the different parts of ourselves in an endless search for meaning: the Third represents our awareness of being pushed in different directions at the same time.

Mary's experience

Mary is a young woman. She is in therapy because of an anxiety disorder that led her to a serious case of somatization: six months of vertigo which prevented her from working and living. She is a rigorous university researcher, recently single after the end of a long, important romantic relationship. Everything in her life went well because her intelligence and effort allowed her to always reach her goals. At one point, however, several of her certainties fell apart: in her straightforward life crops up the shadow of a sudden diagnosis of diabetes; her relationship goes through a crisis. She successfully completes her PhD but fails to take a lighter approach to her post doctorate fellowship. In therapy, she will say that the tragedy for her was having discovered her vulnerability: when this happens, a black liquid fills up her mind. After several rather productive months of individual therapy, Mary joins a group. She recalls the experience as thus:

> *In the beginning I felt extremely embarrassed to have to talk about my experiences and insecurities, but at the same time, I was very curious of my fellow members' troubles. When I told them about my life and my anxiety, I felt a growing empathy coming off of them. Little by little, I started feeling that, in those two hours, time stopped and we were left there telling each other our most intimate fears and thoughts.*
>
> *I discovered that perhaps I was able to see my problems from a different perspective whenever I heard about people having it worse than me, and I found comfort and felt virtually embraced by everyone when I cried because I was in pain.*
>
> *It was a different kind of work from individual therapy, I believe it is a journey of sharing and personal growth that knows no equal: The bond we forge with other members is difficult to break because you showed yourself to them in all your shapes and completely "naked" in their eyes. Perhaps the process of change is slower if compared with individual therapy, but just as valid nonetheless. I will never forget those months and the people I met, with whom I shared an important part of my life, a truly rough patch.*

Acceptance of vulnerability and confrontation with others are factors that introduced in Mary's mind and life the possibility of mediation and the acceptance of the self regardless of performance, thus making her more flexible, more capable of navigating uncertainty.

Toward the end: A stage in itself

In an interesting article, Pinuccia Casalegno (2011) describes the end of therapy as a strategic stage of the therapeutic process with its own goals and strategies of intervention. When the therapist considers the goals, they predict a time and working strategies in order to pursue them.

> A first goal is related to the experiences of separation and the theme of grief that are evoked in the clients by the imminent separation from the therapist. On this matter it is important to encourage the exploration of translational reactions and experiences of deaths, mourning and separations, in order to allow these to be processed and facilitate awareness and perception of any related emotions. In practice, it is important for the client to receive permission to be in touch with themselves, to feel their feelings, without this being perceived as dangerous, so that they might express these feelings safely; we are referring here to the annihilation fantasies connected with the contamination of the Adult by the Child ego state, such as "If I feel pain I might die." A second important aspect consists in encouraging the expression and elaboration of possible negative transferences – such as anger, envy, inferiority and so on, which are connected to separation difficulties. Generally speaking, clients tend to reject these emotions because they are uncomfortable and irritating.
>
> (p. 58)[1]

"I feel ready to end therapy" is the statement that opens the last stage of psychotherapeutic work. A person making this statement is usually ready to confront the therapist and the group. This discussion on which goals were achieved and which were not is particularly rich and allows all group members to reflect on their own journey as well.

"Where am I" is the answer to the stimuli of those who come forward as candidate to the "the end of therapy diploma." This expression is a facetious way to define the end of therapy, qualifying it as a social ritual similar to final high school exams or a bachelor degree, both of which in Italy are government-recognized titles.

When they reach the end of a psychodynamic treatment after a positive confrontation with the group, the client truly feels satisfied and perceives the recognition of the group as a baggage of positive strokes and a blessing from their parents. Peer strokes and blessing from parents make for the necessary fuel to refill the energy quotas of a certain individual, who, at the same time, may also experience the sadness of separation. We can cry together because we will never see each other again, and also lovingly embrace each other one last time; we can miss the nest already, and, at the same time, experience the joy of flying and forging our own path more determinedly and independently than ever.

Often people declare: "I'm saying goodbye because I want to walk on my own two feet." This statement is both true and false. It is false because our clients have always walked on their own feet: after all, they spend with us and the group no more than two hours a week, and do not ask for counsel with regard to every decision they make in the course of their day or week.

It is true, however, that the perception of being in therapy creates in the client's mind an idea of support and dependency that, as it is physiologic, in growing, they wish to eliminate. Thus, putting an end to therapy also acquires a strongly symbolic meaning: I grew as a person, I am an Adult, I left the family house, and I take full responsibility for my life.

When an invitation to end is needed

In the case of clients with dependent disorders, it is often the therapist's job to invite them to end their treatment. There are clients who would never end, if it were up to them. Instead, they would maintain physical closeness to the therapist and the group as some sort of magic protection: "If I stay here, nothing bad can happen to me." The contamination of the Adult ego state by the Child is clearly expressed in these types of statement and can be confronted. More frequently, however, this contamination is not verbalized but acted out.

There was a client, Alex, who used to experience great stress when it came to separating from the group for the summer, and who always had a rough time during the break. Back from vacation, the therapist used to receive a call from Alex in which he introduced himself as if they never met, calling the therapist "doctor," when in group they were on a first name basis. For Alex, each separation represented a loss.

When the moment came for him to put an end to therapy, he said it was not the right moment because he felt very depressed and was experiencing a sudden crisis which allowed him to stay "at home."

Alex was an only child, his father died when he was a teenager and he used to torment his mother asking her to undergo endless check-ups because of his fear she would also get sick and die.

In the same group, Mauro, a client with generalized anxiety disorder and panic attacks, used to ask those who wanted to end therapy a series of questions aimed at demonstrating that they were in fact not ready to end it, and in some cases, he also volunteered to pay another month of therapy because he could not bear the thought of losing that person. Mauro got sick after the fraught separation of his parents, when he was a teenager. When he finally accepted a confrontation on such themes, he had the possibility to live separations in a more constructive manner.

It is thus necessary to confront those who would like to "run away" too early from the process, but also those who would like an endless therapeutic treatment.

Mistakes, fractures, and interruptions

There are situations in which clients and therapists become involved in conflicts, misunderstanding, and ruptures of the alliance in the very final stage of their work. Obviously, in group, everyone has passionate reactions when the end of therapy fails to be agreed-upon and celebrated together. It is difficult to accept that someone wants to "ruin a family party." In such cases, the therapist has to be extremely careful because the client who refuses to satisfy the group's expectations may become the object of a strong hostility from the rest of the group. In the final stage of therapy, people who have troubles with separation and mourning may act out instead of making themselves available to process their feelings, thus leaving conflictual situations unresolved and feelings of anger which would feed the bond instead of break it.

Adele's case

Adele, after manifesting to the group her anger toward the therapist when they failed to validate one of her choices, dropped out and refused to meet the group for the closing sessions expected as per the initial contract. She disappeared from the group angrily, through a few messages to the therapist. Group members were thus unable to talk directly to her and say good-bye. Adele, however, sent each of them a message in which she invited them to dinner so that she could tell her side of the story on the rupture with the therapist, and when everyone refused to meet her outside of the pre-established setting, she became enraged and started accusing all members of being dependent from therapy and too adapted. The therapist became aware of these facts from them.

Adele was an only child with difficult and competitive relationships with her peers, a tendency to provoke and challenge authority and manipulative modes of relation.

When a therapy ends in anger and acting out, it is advisable to ask ourselves, as therapists, what we missed and where we went wrong, and often we discover that we left the client alone precisely when they most needed us. Learning how to separate from others is fundamental in life and it is a skill that can be also strengthened through good modeling in group therapy.

Dropping out without saying goodbye and choosing to disappear is usually a modality that allows clients to avoid feelings related to the intensity of transactional exchanges in a moment of closure. The rituals of the last session, the feedback, and the strokes are all very intense moments and not everyone feels like they can deal with that. The end of therapy for one group member is an important moment of work for all members.

In one of our groups, only after three years, a therapist realized that a client used to always skip the closing session of a leaving member. The therapist finally realized this thanks to an accident: the closing session was postponed to a week later and the avoidant client, in spite of himself, was forced to participate in the final goodbyes, and then confessed his previous flights. The emotional intensity of goodbyes was painful to him and so he always made up excuses not to be there: once he said he had a fever, another time a problem at work, then a toothache and finally a minor car accident.

Failure, trauma, and mourning in group

When in a group someone decides to leave in a tragic way and commits suicide, they involve all members of the group, beside the therapist, in the difficult feat of processing the emotional experiences related to this event. There are people who talk in group about suicide as a way out of depression or even as an experience they had in their family, perhaps a parent who decided to escape the troubles of life that way. It is particularly difficult for the therapist to touch on such a topic in group, as well as to evaluate the risk of giving way to imitations. Despite working in teams integrated with psychiatrists and psychopharmaceutical treatments in cases of severe depression, the risk cannot be avoided completely. In the transactional analysis field, Tony White's (2017) studies are well known and especially relevant to this matter:

> One can have two depressed people side by side with one actively thinking and planning a suicide attempt and the other not even thinking about it or the option of suicide does not even enter his or her thought processes. How can this be explained? The research supports this idea. It shows that around 50% of people with major depression have suicidal ideation and 50% do not (Akechi et al., 2000; Beck, 1967; Wada et al., 1998). How can we explain why 50% of depressed people are suicidal and 50% do not even think of it?
>
> (2017, p. 5)

According to us, it is the presence of the Don't Exist injunction that reveals those truly at risk in stressful situations. White argues:

> Almost everyone at some point has wondered what would it be like to commit suicide, but for those who have not accepted the Don't Exist

injunction, this only remains a fleeting thought and is never seriously considered (Steele & McLennan, 1995). As mentioned earlier, 50% of depressed people have no suicidal ideation. For those who have accepted the Don't Exist injunction, the option of suicidal behavior is very real, and hence, suicidal ideation can become quite influential in the person's decision making.

(2017, p. 6)

Ray Little (2009) explores the psychodynamic reasons that push some clients to commit suicide, and recommends paying special attention to the transference–countertransference matrix in such cases.

Tangolo narrates her experiences on this topic:

Twice in my career as a therapist I have felt a profound hopelessness and my clients in group have been, in turn, great help and comfort to me. When I worked in a therapeutic community, a young man of 20 years old, Mirko, suffered a terrible crisis after having told the group he had been having an incestuous relationship with his alcoholic mother. The boy felt deeply ashamed and he told the group of this tragic experience after his drunken mother had come to the community to take him away. Despite the group's comfort, his shame was so deep that at night he ran away to buy heroin and put an end to a suffering he perceived as unbearable. He was found dead by overdose in the woods.

Many years later, another sweet and fragile client, Achille, at over 40 years old joined a therapy group in order to face the internalized homophobia that led him to hide his homosexuality from everyone and renounce any kind of sexual or romantic life. In group, Achille discovered he could love and be happy, started to frequent the gay scene and began his sexual life. After two years of progress, his mother got severely sick of senile dementia and her care was entrusted to him by his brothers. As a consequence, Achille had a serious depressive breakdown and, despite his treatment being integrated with a pharmacologic treatment and individual therapy, he tried to commit suicide on the very evening he was supposed to have a group session. The paramedics found him just in time and he was admitted to the hospital. Group members went to visit him one by one, but after three days in the hospital he jumped out of a window. This tragic goodbye was very hard on me and the group: we cried together and remembered him with Saint Exupery's words. In our eyes, Achille became the Little Prince we could not convince to stay in our world. The grieving process was long and taxing: within the group, there was a client whose mother died by suicide and another client also had various dramatic experiences of suicide in her

189

family. During this time, I truly understood how difficult and at the same time fundamental it is to be able to accept that we are all together, in group, sharing pain, loss, failure, and trauma. I understood the pain mothers and fathers feel when they lose a child and have to give space to their pain, as well as their siblings', in order to find enough strength to keep living for those who are still alive.

This type of work is very important for the group and we think that, when both members and therapist have to face such a difficult experience, an external support in the form of a supervisor is needed in order to accompany all the steps of the grieving process in which everyone is deeply involved. It is important that the group stay united until members are able to accept other exits and separations, even if of a positive nature and tied to life that goes on.

Through Clara Mucci's (2014) work, we have discovered a text by Judith Butler (2004) which proved especially useful to reflect upon mourning in group. According to Butler, Mucci explains that mourning is not merely a private act, but a political act which recognizes the fundamental relationality of the human being, the very condition for human survival:

> Many people think that grief is privatizing, that it returns us to a solitary situation and is, in that sense, depoliticizing. But I think it furnishes a sense of political community of a complex order, and it does this first of all by bringing to the fore the relational ties that have implications for theorizing fundamental dependency and ethical responsibility. If my fate is not originally or finally separable from yours, then the "we" is traversed by a relationality that we cannot easily argue against.
>
> (Butler, 2004, pp. 22–23)

Each end is a new beginning

The end of therapy does not mean interrupting one's own journey of growth. Those who have known the richness of the group experience usually seek, after ending therapy, group situations in which to spend their free time, such as volunteering or politics, in order to live cultural or affective experiences.

Group sports and organized social experiences are good ways to maintain the rich social life people enjoyed in group therapy. Obviously, according to the different stages of life there are different social exchange needs, but at all age groups are very important in order to be healthy and joyful. For young people, for example, a group is a chance to measure themselves in competition and learning, as well as create romantic and/or sexual relationships.

For people with families, groups are the perfect occasion to compare notes as parents, and have interactions with peers while their kids play together.

For more mature people, too, groups are fundamental moments where to exchange affection and feed their minds. Dance groups, groups centered around card games, or other hobbies clearly demonstrate how these activities improve people's health and resilience until very old age.

Most of all, in all stages of life, the warmth of the group and of friendship are crucial to human life.

Notes on healing

The ideas related to healing, change, maturation, and health are connected to our perspective on life and human beings. On this particular matter, psychology must inevitably join forces with philosophy and the human sciences. To give only few examples, we can employ different definitions of "healing" to guide both therapists and clients during treatment.

Yalom and Leszcz (2005) write that people are never cured, they merely change or grow (p. 14). Nonetheless, the term "healing" carries its own beauty and meaning. We let clients define the result of their journey as healing, growth or change. One group member declared he had been "healed as much as possible" meaning that each person has in mind a possible balanced state for themselves, thus empowering the subject to define their own goals.

Berne (1972) talked about providing clients with a fishing license (p. 123), that is, "a license to give up behavior which the Adult wants to give up, or a release from negative behavior" (p. 375).

Thinking about a hypothetical client, Berne (1966) also added that:

> The reason he can "cured" is that while one part of him clings to the Santa Claus fantasy and would rather live in a fairy tale world than give up hope, some other part of him knows that it is an illusion. . . .
> The therapist can offer him the whole real world to replace the lost illusion – new lamps for old nostalgias, a fresh red apple for the vanished orb.
>
> Transactionally what actually happens in this framework is as follows: the patient comes to the therapist with the idea that the therapist has the patient's cure at his disposal, probably locked in his desk. It is only because the therapist is demanding, stingy, mean, or selfish that he does not hand it to the patient immediately at the first interview, but the patient has little doubt at first that if he behaves well enough for long enough, it will be given to him, very much as Santa Claus would give him presents when he was little.

(pp. 284–285)

Tangolo (2010/2015) writes that:

> For most people, healing means growing up, giving up their childish illusions and demands and managing to get by in the "grown-up" world by their own efforts and thanks to the support of other, a support exchanged on the basis of a principle of mutuality.
>
> Mutuality means relationships in which giving and taking are balanced and imply free choice and the possibility of also making gifts.
>
> Healing thus means accepting the human condition of being-in-the-world, of existing, of being thrown into the world, of being able to make projects within boundaries that are not completely determined by us, like our birth and our death, as described by Heidegger (1962).
>
> (p. 138)

In an interesting article, Tudor (2016) writes on the therapist's duty to provide permission, protection, and potency according to Berne's model, in order to facilitate the client's healing:

> Just as a license does not compel one to fish, a permission does not compel one to challenge the injunction or resolve the impasse. Berne also added three ideas to the concept of permission. First, there are negative permissions: Whereas the positive permission cuts off the injunction, the negative permission (e.g., "Stop pushing him into it") cuts off the provocation. Second, permission is, or can be, the cure (e.g., "The cure for the scriptless aged is permission"). Third, in a section on the dynamics of permission, he suggested a more complex permission diagram.
>
> (2016, p. 53)

> Writing about protection, Berne (1972) clearly linked it to potency: The therapist should feel potent enough to deal with the patient's Parent and "the patient's Child must believe he [the therapist] is potent enough, to offer protection from the Parental wrath" (p. 374). Berne also wrote that the therapist's protective power "resides as much in the timbre of his voice as in what he says" (p. 375) and diagrammed it as a Parent-Child transaction in the context of the overall permission transaction.
>
> (2016, p. 56)

A client ending therapy in a constructive and shared way with group and therapist feels like they have internalized the possibility of going in that same direction of growth and health. The inner Parent can thus provide the three P's: Permission, Protection, and Potency.

Note

1 My translation.

References

Akechi, T., Okamura, H., Kugaya, A., Nakano, T., Nakanishi, T., Akizuki, N., . . . Uchitomi, Y. (2000). Suicidal ideation in cancer patients with major depression. *Japanese Journal of Clinical Oncology, 30*, 221–224.

Beck, A. T. (1967). *Depression: Clinical, experimental, and theoretical aspects.* London: Staples Press.

Benjamin, J. (2017). *Beyond doer and done to: Recognition theory, intersubjectivity and the third.* London and New York: Routledge.

Berne, E. (1966). *Principles of group treatment.* Oxford: Oxford University Press.

Berne, E. (1972). *What do you say after you say hello?: The psychology of human destiny.* New York: Bantam Books.

Butler, J. (2004). *Precarious life: The powers of mourning and violence.* London and New York: Verso.

Casalegno, P. (2011). La conclusione come fase strategica della terapia. *Neopsiche, 10.*

Heidegger, M. (1962). *Being and time.* New York: Harper & Row (Originally published in 1927).

Little, R. (2009). Understanding the psychodynamics of suicidal clients: Exploring suicidal and presuicidal states. *Transactional Analysis Journal, 39*, 219–228. doi:10.1177/036215370903900305

Luborsky, L., & Crits-Christoph, P. (1990). *Understanding transference: The core conflictual relationship theme method.* New York: Basic Books.

Mucci, C. (2014). *Trauma e perdono.* Milano: Raffaello Cortina.

Steele, A. A., & McLennan, J. (1995). Suicidal and counter-suicidal thinking. *Australian Psychologist, 30*, 149–152. doi:10.1080/00050069508258921

Tangolo, A. E. (2015). *Psychodynamic psychotherapy with transactional analysis: Theory and narration of a living experience* (A. Iozzelli & K. Jones, Trans.). London: Karnac (Originally published in 2010).

Tudor, K. (2016). Permission, protection, and potency. *Transactional Analysis Journal, 46*(1), 50–62. doi:10.1177/0362153715617475

Wada, K., Murao, J., Hikasa, K., Ota, T., Kinoshita, S., & Yoshinari, H. (1998). A clinical analysis of the suicidal ideation of outpatients with major depression. *Sheishin Igaku, 39*, 1077–1082.

White, T. (2017). A transactional analysis perspective on suicide risk assessment. *Transactional Analysis Journal, 47*(1), 32–41. doi:10.1177/0362153716674683

Yalom, I. D., & Leszcz, M. (2005). *The theory and practice of group psychotherapy.* New York: Basic Books (Originally published in 1970).

18

A CASE STUDY

A necessary preface

Describing group processes is akin to writing a film script and, as the written text is not the same as a movie, the description of a group process is not the same as the process itself.

In order to understand how a group functions, we have to dive deep inside the environment generated by transactions and looks, and experience firsthand the extraordinary closeness that this context manages to create. What we are trying to do here is to describe a piece of a conversation as it happened in a group therapy session. The narration that follows was created by the therapist and subsequently read and discussed by the actual group, with clients giving their consent for publication. Our aim is to illustrate the complexity and the intensity of the first few minutes of the session: The transition from a state of solitary reflection to one of sociality, which leads quickly – as Berne (1964) would say – from isolation to pastimes and games.

Following Wilma Bucci's (1997) example, we could describe group therapy as an attempt to verbalize a non-verbal experience – symbolic and sub-symbolic – in which the therapist must strengthen the referential process in order to lead the clients' mind-bodies toward an integration of their split parts. Another way of describing it could entail focusing on some therapeutic factors typical of the group context, such as those previously cited and delineated by Yalom's (2009) theory. Alternatively, we could interview the individual group members so as to study the core conflictual relationships according to Luborsky and Christoph's (1990) model.

In summary, the strong intensity and high complexity of the group experience allow for it to be described from many different points of view, and open up several research directions. As therapists, the path we would like to take is the one we have already stated: exposing the clients' recurring emotional patterns thus making them aware of these, and experimenting together with new patterns and models within an open and generative environment.

DOI: 10.4324/9781003215547-19

The first 15 minutes of a group session, scripted

Characters

First therapist, Anna Emanuela, 56 years old: A transactional analyst, has been leading group sessions for more than 20 years. She oversees these clients' training and therapy.

Second therapist, Sherouk, 40 years old: A cognitivist psychotherapist, training in transactional analysis. After completing her theoretical training on group therapy, a year ago she started co-leading this group.

Licia, 56 years old: A referral by a colleague of Anna Emanuela, who is seeing her in individual sessions. She is a very smart, single woman, graduated in pharmacy. She has been in therapy for many years due to her bipolar disorder, and she is currently out of a job after quitting to take care of her mother, who died around three years ago. She gained some weight because of antidepressants, she feels lonely but says she is incapable of maintaining romantic or friendly relationships, she engages in catastrophic thinking. In the beginning, she was often hostile and aggressive toward others. At times, she expresses her need for affection, only to become overly critical and push away any help offered to her.

Ciro, 51 years old: Has a long psychiatric history of anxiety, OCD, and depression, as well as a very heavy family history. His alcoholic father died when he was a teenager. His mother suffered from a severe case of paranoid disorder and killed herself when Ciro was 35. His older sister died of brain cancer shortly after his mother's suicide. He is married, with a ten-year-old son, and works as a government employee. Through psychotherapy, he managed to suppress all symptoms and live ten peaceful years, but, approaching 50, a year after finishing treatment, he relapsed into depression and asked to go back to the group.

Mario, 40 years old: A physiotherapist, joined the group after a psychoanalytical therapy that aimed at confronting his affective ambivalence toward women. He has a 12-year-old daughter, and has been in a very unhappy relationship for four years with a woman whom he cannot let go of and yet, cannot accept as a life partner. He has at times a very passionate relationship with this woman, despite the fact that she rejects him sexually and treats him like a traitor even though he has never actually hurt her deliberately. He feels everyday more involved and unhappy.

Marina, 35 years old: A psychologist, came to the group after a few years of individual therapy for training purposes. She is married, with two teenage daughters, and comes from the south of Italy, which she left for work-related reasons. She suffers from dysthymic disorder. She has improved in dealing with her depressive crises, but she remains restless and feels frequently unsatisfied with her social and affective life. Her relationship with her family of origin is fraught with conflict, since she feels rejected and excluded by them. Faced with competition and the risk to arouse or feel envy, she prefers withdrawal and isolation.

Delia, 37 years old: A psychologist, she joined the group in order to complete her training. She has two young children and a husband very attached to his career who tends to enable her tendency to fall into the role of Cinderella. An only child of a small, middle class, northern family, she often feels isolated and misunderstood. She had undertaken an important course of study which she interrupted to become a full time mother.

Lily, 44 years old: A pedagogist, she joined the group because of intense loneliness. She lives with her husband and a much-beloved four-year-old daughter. Her general attitude toward life is of a phobic type. She is slow to change and tends to be dependent on people, especially her husband.

Sonia, 45 years old: An educator, she came back to group therapy many years after finishing a previous treatment. This she started because of a pervasive anxiety disorder, which surfaced after having entered in a relationship with a former drug addict. She went back to therapy after separating from her husband, a chronic alcoholic, who developed a serious psychiatric disorder. While she is in therapy, her husband dies. She is raising her teenage daughter on her own.

A methodological preface and some information

This group has been meeting every Thursday night for many years. The maximum number of participants is eight. When someone ends their treatment and leaves the group, someone else can join. Thus, in this type of setting, somebody who has just started treatment may find an already formed group in which some members have been in the group for two years and others a few months. The newcomers see the group as a solid organism and experience their own entry like a true initiation ritual, strongly and emotionally charged with all those fantasies and projections which, according to Berne, make up the "provisional group imago": when members join the group, they imagine it as their family of origin, and give the therapist a parental role (transference slot). They also fantasize about being treated by others the same way they were in fact treated during their first social entry into the world.

Longtime members can experience this arrival in different ways, depending on the reactions to change and novelty that are built into their scripts, as well as on the specific therapy stage they are going through. People who have been in the group for a long time are undergoing a period of relearning and approaching the end of treatment they often welcome with pleasure a new "sibling" to which they can "pass on the baton," so to speak, share their experience and recount their journey, and are curious to know what the newcomer brings with them in terms of knowledge and affectivity. For those in this conclusive stage being part of a big group means receiving more affection, having a wider audience, living in a context that's richer in terms of life, happiness, and pain – in short, a higher intensity of interactions. Those who are still in the storming stage, on the contrary, will show hostility toward therapist and group when faced with this change, expressing it both explicitly and passively, displaying withdrawal behaviors and making attempts at excluding the newcomer, such as talking about topics the newly arrived can't understand without giving any explanation.

Finally, those who are going through the operative group imago phase, where game are more present, will give the newcomer a warm welcome on the surface, but will soon start trying to hook them into games of seduction and aggressive provocation. Unwittingly following their scripts, they will seek in these games a sadistic satisfaction, hoping to find in the newcomer an easy prey or an onlooker.

In light of these first few considerations, we can understand how portraying a group is no easy feat. In fact, it means offering a sample in which what happens to everyone is shown as experienced by each individual member in a different way, also depending on the various therapeutic stages they are at. If each of them told their own version of the same session, we could listen to many different stories as if in a modernist novel with several points of view, in which the story is fragmented and then recollected in a concerted narration that is the product of many distinct voices. The polyphonic character of groups has yet to be researched by scientific literature. On the other hand, it is well documented in fiction, for example in *The Schopenhauer Cure* (2009), a novel by Irvin D. Yalom, where, nonetheless, the narrating voice remains that of the therapist. An attempt at group description which might open new research directions should, in our opinion, take as a model a polyphonic composition, a play, or a story in which there is no unique narrating voice, as it happens, for example, in *The Lover (1977)*, the famous novel by A. B. Yehoshua. Here, every character expresses themselves in a first-person point of view through long or short monologues (at times full of inner dialogues related to what they are thinking or experiencing). Yehoshua himself, in his book *Il lettore allo specchio: Sul romanzo e la scrittura* (2003), recounts how he wrote *The Lover* with apprehension, dealing for the first time with fiction thanks to the theatre:

> Writing about it allowed me to free myself from the first person, from the narrator, that is usually the point around which all characters gravitate. So I was able to put everyone on the same level. Yet, I still hesitated because in order to write a novel it is necessary to have a clear vision of the kind of society you want to depict. It was during that time that I discovered Faulkner, *The Sound and the Fury* and *As I Lay Dying*, to be exact. In these novels I found that monologues may be intertwined to form a polyphony, a novel of many voices.
>
> (Yehoshua & Guetta, 2003, p. 53)[1]

Just before the start of the session

Licia

I'm a bit late, as usual. I don't like going out at this hour, leaving my dog alone. I put on my sandals, they feel tight on my swollen feet. The lipstick makes me feel even more awkward and ridiculous. I don't know why I'm even going, the others must be there already. Tonight I feel like fighting, if Ciro is there he'll surely say something stupid. That'll give me the chance to tell him off. And anyway, last Thursday he didn't offer me a glass of water and was making eyes at Marina. He only does that because she's younger and complains all the time (I can't stand her).

Ciro is nice, but he has to stop pushing me to find a job. If he tells me one more time to write up a CV, I swear I'll scream at him. I hope Delia's there, a friendly face at least.

Why do I even keep going?

Ciro

It's seven o'clock, I finished work an hour ago but I can't stop thinking about that damn case. Maybe I should take the case files home on Saturday so I can work on it some more during the weekend. I'm not going to be able to catch up even by December. But I haven't eaten yet and the usual pizzeria is closed, what should I do? I don't know where to go now, I can't try a new place tonight, I'm too exhausted. I'll just get a cappuccino at the bar, today I didn't even take a break. Thankfully, the group is tonight. I just want to sit down with them, I don't have a lot to say, I just need company. I hope Licia is not too harsh on me tonight, I'm too tired to respond. Although, sometimes I almost appreciate her attacks, I feel seen by her. After all, her remarks are always very smart, it's my fault I never know what to say. I don't know why I keep going there, I just know it makes me feel better, and that if I don't go, I feel a great emptiness. Maybe that's why I relapsed after the end of my last treatment. Emptiness, I'm scared of the great emptiness.

Mario

I'm in a hurry, as usual, but why am I in a hurry to go to therapy? I thought I was going to therapy to learn how to relax? Maybe I shouldn't have come tonight, it's too much pressure, I'll say I work too much, that I can't go every week anymore, that I need a break, a leave of absence, they'll understand, they'll accept it. Truth is, I don't have the guts to tell them I had sex with Maria again, after I told them so proudly that I'd ended it last week, and they were so supportive of that "healthy" decision. I don't know if I want to be healthy: If she calls me I go nuts, even tonight I was looking for an excuse to go to her. But she disappeared, as usual: When I give in to her she likes to play the tyrant. I can't tell the truth. I'll try to let the others speak, be quiet, this time I'm too ashamed. I feel like I'm the dumb one, the one who's always starting from scratch, who's always back to square one, who never achieves a thing. The therapists are quiet, but I can feel their contempt. I'd love for them to appreciate me, to respect me, but maybe I don't even respect myself. I feel the same way I felt when, as a kid, I used to shit myself and pretend nothing happened until the smell enveloped me completely.

Marina

I don't know if I should stay in the group. I need more attention, maybe I could try psychoanalysis, but I have to find a woman as therapist, someone who's able to finally see me. This group feels exactly like my family, they never see me, I don't get the same attention as everybody else. For example, Anna Emanuela follows Mario very closely, she allows him things she doesn't allow me. How come I'm never important enough?

Delia

Today I can say I feel better, but I'm never really happy. Is this because of my past traumas? It's my husband's absence, I realize more and more he only sees himself. I need him to see me, to love me. I feel like he only used me as mother of his children, I don't know, I don't know.

Lily

Thanks to this treatment I was able to get my driving license, but it's all so exhausting to me! I don't know if they can understand that. Even now I'm going to the meeting by bus and I asked my husband to come pick me up after, and I'm ashamed to tell them. I don't feel comfortable driving at night, I don't feel safe and I feel like everyone expects too much of me. I won't say anything, I just hope nobody sees me coming.

Sonia

I get Mario, he's lucky to have someone to spend his nights with. I can't stand sleeping in that cold, empty bed anymore. I know they'll tell me the bed was already empty because sometimes he didn't come back to sleep, because he came back drunk and high at six in the morning, but at least there was still hope for him to come back then, for me to feel his warm body next to mine. At least I could fool myself into thinking something could change, at least. It's hard to admit that during the day you're a strong, resolute, admirable woman, but at night you fall apart and don't recognize yourself in that loneliness, in the loss of that dream. Even when it comes to the group, I feel good when we're all there, sitting close to each other on the sofas, in the warmth of the living room and of our interactions, having the kind of loving and affectionate conversations I can never have with anybody else. At night, though, the group becomes a ghost that judges me when I feel nostalgic about the past.

Anna Emanuela (first therapist)

We start in half an hour. Tonight I'm tired, it was a hard week, I can't think about the lady who was in that terrible accident; maybe I should visit her in the hospital.

But I'm so tired, I was looking forward to Friday to take some time off. Sometimes I feel like I'm drowning in all the demands, phone calls, and other people's needs. Tonight, with the group, I'd like to sit down and just talk, I'd like for them to be all there for me. Maybe I should go back to therapy or at least work less.

Sherouk (second therapist)

I'm a bit late, when I go from one studio to the other I'm always a little nervous. I like this experience, I'm learning so much from group therapy. Co-leading this group is, for me, an incredible training ground, so I'm very happy I was accepted into this program, which is not easy at all. It feels like weaving on a mysterious loom, or preparing a recipe that I don't know the ingredients for. I don't think I can afford to follow closely the interweaving of eight simultaneous treatments, and, at the same time, give in to a surprising and creative improvisation, like my colleague does. It is something that goes beyond my present abilities. I've been doing this for a year now, but they told me that it takes at least three years to have any idea on how to lead a therapy group.

8:30 pm, the session starts

When people come in and sit down to start the meeting, everyone has already activated an inner monologue which includes memories from previous meetings and interpretations of past experiences and social interactions, filtered through their own defensive scripts. In a way, each member comes into the group still having this inner monologue, that is finally interrupted by real personal exchanges. Leaving this isolation leads, according to Berne, first to a series of stereotypical interactions, rituals, which are then followed by pastimes. Pastimes may seem trivial and filling, but they are actually used to throw hooks and look for partners willing to participate in psychological games. During these games, we enact our scripts hoping to finally find the love and social recognition we missed out on in the past, but actually end up subconsciously looking for and finding once again a confirmation of our disappointed expectations, to which follow regret and resignation.

Only if these games are exposed, we can then move on toward constructive social interactions and the much-coveted intimacy, which happens solely when we are able to be our authentic selves amidst other authentic selves: Many true "I"s, capable of becoming an "us."

*

Everyone has arrived at the meeting, except Licia who will get there ten minutes later.

CIRO: Where's Licia? I'm a bit worried about her, I'm afraid I offended her last session when I offered to help her with her CV again.

SONIA: You're too pushy and you never know when to shut up, last week was definitely not a good moment to bring up her CV. I would have killed you.

LILY: What happened? Why isn't Licia coming?

FIRST THERAPIST: Licia didn't say anything about her absence tonight, so I encourage you all to talk about this when she comes in. It's better to share your worries with her and tell her you're afraid of having hurt her, Ciro.

DELIA: Ciro, you have directly to talk to her.

MARINA: Wait for her to come, you need to have this exchange with her.

CIRO: All right, I'll wait, but I felt really bad about it and I even tried to call her but she didn't pick up.

SONIA: See, you always put yourself first, I, I, I . . . if it's really her you're thinking about, wait, shut up and let's see if you can learn to be a little more empathetic toward others, since your timing is always off.

SECOND THERAPIST: Right now you, Sonia, are telling Ciro some important things, but in a very critical way. . .

Licia comes in, slamming the door

LICIA: Hello everyone, have you started already?

DELIA: Yes, a few minutes ago and we were just talking about you. . .

MARIO: Don't worry, it's just that Ciro felt guilty about what he told you last Thursday and he was afraid you weren't coming.

LICIA: If he feels guilty then good for him, but he does not have that much power over me!

FIRST THERAPIST: If there's something you want to tell each other than do it openly.

CIRO: I'm sorry, I think I was careless and I hurt you.

LICIA: I was crying, for me it was as if you weren't understanding my problems at all and were just twisting the knife. I know I should be looking for a job too, but I'm ashamed, at my age it's not easy to start from scratch.

DELIA: I can help you if you want.

LICIA: The thing is, that makes me feel even more stupid. I'm not here to get material help, but to feel understood and find enough strength in myself to do things.

FIRST THERAPIST: It seems to me that now you're all speaking from a deeper place: You, Licia, about your problems and your shame, and you, Ciro, about your regret because you realized you were out of synch with Licia and your attempt at being there for her was a bit of a blunder to her.

CIRO: Yes, my wife used to tell me all the time I didn't understand her feelings either, but at least now I'm trying. . .

MARINA: We have to give that to him! He always makes an effort, with all of us.

CIRO: Thanks, Marina, you're always on my side.

FIRST THERAPIST: And what does that mean to you, Ciro?

CIRO: I'm surprised, it's something new. It's never happened to me before, not at home, not as a boy, and not even as a father and husband. It feels good to have someone who understands and supports you.

LICIA: By the way, we're still talking about him, always about him. Boring!

SECOND THERAPIST: What is it that irritates you, Licia?

LICIA: I don't know, I don't know. Maybe it's the same thing that happens with my brother, it feels like he's always taking space from me, even when he wants to help. And he's so trite, always stating the obvious, our Ciro.

CIRO: I knew she would drag me into it again. . . [smiling, pleased he was mentioned].

SECOND THERAPIST: Well, Licia, don't start berating Ciro again. I encourage you to think about what you were saying before about the space that Ciro might be taking away from you, the same way your brother did in the past. So is it a defensive mechanism that you're reproducing?

LICIA: Yes, I always attack those who threaten to steal space and attentions from me.

FIRST THERAPIST: It's important you realize that you're using the words "threat" and "thief" to define someone who speaks the way Ciro does.

LICIA: You're right, I might be biased . . . I'm always so cruel to my friend Giulio and he always forgives me.

FIRST THERAPIST: That's still an aggressive behavior that might make other people push you away.

LICIA: [Sighing] It happens often.

SECOND THERAPIST: Is that what you want? To be left alone? To make everyone run away?

LICIA: I always complain I'm lonely, I get it, unless I change something, I'm the cause of my own loneliness.

MARINA: [To the therapists] Is this a game, this one Licia is playing with Ciro?

FIRST THERAPIST: What do you think?

MARIO: Of course, what is astonishing is the way it always repeats itself in the same way. It's very similar to what happens to me with Maria. Even if I see it, I can't do anything to stop it.

DELIA: If understanding were enough, the treatment would be so short!

CIRO: Then what is it supposed to happen for us to heal?

LICIA: For you healing would look like finally dropping the useless platitudes and expressing your feelings.

CIRO: And for you it would look like not being so nasty with everyone anymore.

MARINA: Don't start bickering again, I think it's more important here to understand how to really change things, since almost all of us here are caught up in the same cycles.

CIRO: You mean the scripts.

SONIA: [Ironically] Great, Ciro! You don't speak much, but when you do, you say such brilliant things.

MARINA: Can we go back to what I said before? How can we truly, deeply change?

FIRST THERAPIST: Is it an explanation you need, Marina? [she nods]

All right, so, let's say that what needs to change lies with an internal relationship that we'll call the Parent–Child relation [drawing on the board]. Until the inner Parent embraces appropriately the Child's needs, change doesn't happen. But also, until the inner Child experiences the benefit of growing up, change doesn't last. Have you experienced or observed any lasting changes in the group?

*

At the end of this exchange, Marina feels reassured by the explanation received and because she managed to insert herself in an interaction she was initially excluded from. This is very important for her.

Licia managed to stir everyone's interest but, after an initial position of rejection and hostility toward Ciro-her brother, she also opened up to a constructive exchange.

Ciro was able to experience different emotional reactions to his behavior and found a way to make amends for his lack of empathy toward Licia thanks to the others' affection and understanding, Marina especially.

Delia managed to say something, making an attempt at existing inside the group, as did Lily, who still kept mostly to the sidelines.

Mario finds a way to tell the group he went back on his decision to break up with Maria. He manages to do it without feeling too ashamed, by referring to other members' relapses into their own script activations.

Conclusions

We have just described a few minutes of a group therapy session. We would like to point out to the reader the complexity of the interactions in this brief section. In particular, it is interesting to note how the repetitive and predictable elements of scripted transactions (the ulterior transactions which are at the basis of dysfunctional games) are interspersed with little elements of novelty, marked by small changes in the transactions. The apparently modest extent of these changes should not be misleading: as with nautical routes, a variation of a few degrees at sea is enough to lead the ship to a completely different harbor.

In this example, we saw how the group functions as a place of projection in which clients enact their family scripts. After acknowledging the limits of the repetitive dynamics, this place allows them to go through a corrective experience of interpersonal learning. This will acquire more and more meaning and value as the clients experiment with the possibility to change course and attest the benefits that follow.

The conflict between their need for the certainty and predictability of social transactions and the desire to fulfill in a deeper way their need for intimacy and love can be fully expressed within the group. This conflict may engender a harsh confrontation at times and may manifest itself as a literal war of likes and dislikes, but all members accept it knowing that others often represent rejected part of themselves.

At the end of Yalom's novel (2009), when a new group is born, we can read this excellent exchange between the two leaders and the new members:

"Wait, wait, let's freeze the action for a moment," said Tony, "and get some feedback on our first five minutes from the other members here. First, I want to say something to you, Jason, and to you, Marsha – something that Philip and I learned from Julius, our teacher. Now, I'm sure you two feel like this is a stormy beginning but I've got a hunch, a very strong hunch, that by the end of this group, each of you are going to prove very valuable to the other. Right, Philip?"

"Right you are, partner."

(p. 365)

Note

1 My translation.

References

Berne, E. (1964). *Games people play: The psychology of human relationships*. New York: Grove Press.

Bucci, W. (1997). Symptoms and symbols: A multiple code theory of somatization. *Psychoanalytic Inquiry, 17*(2), 151–172. doi:10.1080/07351699709534117

Luborsky, L., & Crits-Christoph, P. (1990). *Understanding transference: The core conflictual relationship theme method*. New York: Basic Books.

Yalom, I. D. (2009). *The Schopenhauer cure*. New York: Harper Perennial.

Yehoshua, A. B. (1977). *The Lover* (P. Simpson, Trans.). New York: Doubleday.

Yehoshua, A. B., & Guetta, A. (2003). *Il lettore allo specchio: Sul romanzo e la scrittura*. Torino: Einaudi.

19

ONLINE GROUPS AT THE TIME OF CORONAVIRUS

An ongoing case study

A premise

All over the world, therapists have been using an online therapeutic setting for a few years now, but it really depends on the local culture and the degree of digitalization of the different countries.

The widespread usage of social networks in the last decade and the revolution that was web 2.0 has deeply changed the work and life habits of millions of people. It is considerably easier now to find people who can communicate through Skype with their relatives on the other side of the world, use WhatsApp even without adequate digital literacy and meet on Facebook, Tinder, or whichever new meeting app. We employ social networks to reunite with family, make new friends, have sex, and buy all kinds of things.

In this context, telemedicine has improved significantly over the years, providing better access to health care services to many people and communities with geographical barriers. Online psychology and psychotherapeutic treatment have had for many years their own specific protocols and consensus from scientific associations and health care insurance companies. Groups are among the latest forms of therapy to be accepted and tested without contraindications, even though, obviously, it depends on the technological systems that can guarantee at once security and efficiency.

In the English-speaking world and the United States, this type of experience is more well established, as are the legal and ethical protocols related to the use of the Internet in psychotherapy. In Europe, interest in this field has emerged only recently, and the circumstances of the 2020 pandemic forced all clients and therapists to approach the world of telemedicine and online psychology.

In an interesting article published in the third edition of Fehr's (2018) handbook on group therapy, Shari Baron (2018) traces the history of the American cultural context, in which great associations such as APA and the group therapy association worked together to delineate the ethical and legal protocols of online therapy. In her definition:

> Telepsychology describes individual or group practice consisting of ongoing synchronous or asynchronous conversations in which the client,

DOI: 10.4324/9781003215547-20

therapist and other group members are in separate or remote locations
and utilize electronic means to communicate with each other.

(Baron, 2018, p.276)

In the English-speaking world, great attention has been given to the legal and
ethical issues arising from these new types of setting. The APA has defined since
2013 the framework in which therapist has to operate and the concerns that must
be paramount in tele-psychology.

*

While we are writing, the coronavirus outbreak has taken the world by storm, with
dire consequences on everyone's lives – among these, in Italy as in many other
parts of the world, lockdown, suspension of all social gatherings and mandatory
social distancing. An aftereffect of these restrictive measures is the change in how
psychotherapy is carried out, since the only way it can be practiced at the present
moment is online, through the different video conferencing and chat platforms
offered by the Internet. Therapists and clients alike have had to deal with this new
setting, which, given the present circumstances, is the only way to allow the meeting to be a safe space and a secure opportunity for treatment.

Group therapy represented the real challenge in these strange times. Many
therapists suspended their clinical group activity thinking that social distancing
would be a brief, temporary measure, and that all practices and clinics would have
soon reopened.

Unfortunately, that was not the case, and social gatherings are still forbidden
as we write.

As certified TSTA professionals, in our centers in Tuscany and the rest of Italy,
we promote and supervise more than 60 therapy groups led by an equal number
of therapists, and in the animated discussions of the first few weeks of emergency,
we chose to start right away experimenting with online group therapy.

Several American associations, in time, produced some studies and documents
about telemedicine and the use of internet in psychotherapy (AMA, 2000; APA,
1997, 2012; ATA, 2009a, 2009b, 2010).

As early as 2012, in a research about videoconference in psychotherapy, Backhaus, Agha and Maglione stated:

The results indicate that VCP is feasible, has been used in a variety of
therapeutic formats and with diverse populations, is generally associated with good user satisfaction, and is found to have similar clinical
outcomes to traditional face-to-face psychotherapy.

(Backhaus et al., 2012)

In Italy, however, the digitalization process of many activities is still very much
behind compared to the United States and many European countries, in regard to
both the technological resources and social acceptance of it.[1] In light of this, we

206

have indeed encountered a fair amount of resistance from clients and therapists alike.[2]

At the beginning, the clients' most frequent objections were: *I don't have an internet connection at home, how do I isolate myself from my family and have enough privacy to join the therapy session? I'm not good with technology, I think it's a very cold way to communicate.*

From the therapists' point of view, the most common objections were: *I cannot see my clients clearly, I can't see their whole bodies, I can't connect emotionally with them, I'm not good with technology, if somebody refuses this change of setting I won't be able to move forward.*

While supervising, we examined the different objections by clients and therapists and we found that often they turned out to be what in TA is called a "double contamination," resulting in prejudices and phobias.

A Parent contamination of the Adult results in prejudices and generalizations, such as the belief that in order to communicate effectively, it is necessary to see each other in person. A Child contamination of the Adult results in illusions and phobias, for example, with respect to the Internet or that "magical object" that is a smartphone and its video calls. This way, as it were, clients who thought they did not have an internet connection, in many cases had a smartphone and a telephone plan with several gigabytes of data which, until that moment, they had used exclusively for things such as Facebook and other social media that now enjoy a high degree of popularity in Italy across all generations. Our recommendation to therapists was that they talk to their clients – suggesting they download a video conferencing app – and that they organize a trial group, supported by a group chat on a messaging app, to be used in case of technical difficulties. In the space of two weeks, everyone acquired the knowledge and competences needed to make or join video calls, and thus, we reinstated group therapy sessions, as per the original schedule. At that point, therapists were very surprised to notice that all groups had resumed their scheduled activities with an insignificant percentage of premature terminations and with some interesting differences. We were expecting to lead emotional support groups to face fears related to the pandemic, social distancing and anxiety due to the incumbent economic crisis, and of course these were common discussion topics, but what was truly surprising was seeing emotional interactions that were deeper and more intense than we had imagined. Behind the apparent barrier of a computer screen or a smartphone, people share their day-to-day fears with intense emotion: crying is not inhibited and clients fully express their anxieties, anger and sadness at being separated from their loved ones. Moreover, we found that often dreams came up spontaneously in members' accounts, dreams in which therapists and other members make explicit appearances. This seemed to confirm the depth of the therapeutic work being done and the clients' emotional openness.

Individuals who are generally more reserved or inhibited, avoidant, or obsessive were the ones most at ease from the very beginning, and encouraged others to communicate like never before. People who live alone found great comfort in the weekly sessions, they let us enter their living rooms, they showed us their cats or dogs, they eagerly await every session. Young mothers with toddlers could take a moment away from their children, who, despite their greed for the mother's time, were left in the care of partners during group sessions. Teenagers, scared by a lack of privacy, retired in the safety of their cars in order to participate. Only a few clients suffering from borderline personality disorder occasionally found fertile ground for new games, such as leaving the call and then joining again with an excuse about having connectivity problems, so as to compensate the impossibility of astonishing everyone with their usual "scenes" and "fireworks," which through a screen appeared duller and flatter.

The experiment will continue because of necessity, maybe even for several more months until the world will be able to return to a new normal. As therapists, we have learnt that it is possible to conduct online therapy groups and thus we could add to our regular therapeutic tools also groups working entirely in an online setting. We are certain technology will come to our aid more and more providing firm support to meetings. Clients who live thousands of kilometers away from each other will then be able to join, and group therapy will be available to many more people, from individuals who live with different forms of disabilities to those who live and work far away from city centers, in places that are hard to reach but are now connected to the world through the internet.

In a recent study, Norwood and others affirm:

> Videoconferencing psychotherapy (VCP) – the remote delivery of psychotherapy via secure video link – is an innovative way of delivering psychotherapy, which has the potential to overcome many of the regularly cited barriers to accessing psychological treatment. However, some debate exists as to whether an adequate working alliance can be formed between therapist and client, when therapy is delivered through such a medium.
>
> (Norwood, Moghaddam, Malins, & Sabin-Farrell, 2018, p. 1)

To be sure, more evidence has still to be provided in order to solve these doubts. In this respect, we would like to share some of our current experiences with online group therapy, hoping in so doing to nurture this stimulating conversation.

An experience of emotional support

The group, led by two therapists, meets on Tuesday nights. It is composed by eight people and among them only Anna (45 years old, office worker) refuses to continue the work online because she lives alone with a teenage son and is scared she won't have enough privacy.

Gina (60 years old, physiotherapist) initially rejects the idea of online sessions on the grounds that she lives in a remote country area with sparse internet connectivity. Elena (50 years old, shop assistant) follows suit saying she is not good with technology and will wait for the in-person sessions to start again.

Antonio (50 years old) is a manager used to work remotely and doesn't have any problems with the online setting, as Gianni (52 years old), an entrepreneur who's not afraid of the new challenge but, on the contrary, seems curious.

Luca (29 years old) is a young researcher also used to work remotely and he regards this arrangement as particularly favorable, since it allows him to continue the group work while living in another city, where he spends a lot of his time.

Neither Miriam nor Luisa (30 years old, respectively, student and office worker), two independent young women used to working and studying from home and using social networks, have any problem with the online setting. So, among conflicting opinions, the group begins its online activity and from the second session on Gina and Elena decide to join as well, discovering excitedly a new way of communication.

Gina is about to retire. She is getting ready to enter a new stage of her life and found herself stuck in the house just as she could finally travel. She brings her eagerness into the group recounting her dreams:

I'm at a tram stop, or any other kind of stop. There are two young men with two little girls and I'm with my sister Maria [only a few months dead].

We can read here the representation of the group that follows her in her transformation process. Gina's dreams present a variety of scenarios, from exciting adventures to familiar places and habits: The cup of coffee in the usual coffee shop, the bakery where one of the two young men offers her some fresh bread, the warm colors dominating the scenery. When she wakes up, she feels in a good mood.

Elena is caring for her mother suffering from terminal-stage brain cancer, and is experiencing a period of illness and grief.

In the midst of the pandemic, Miriam and Luisa's studies and work seem to have come to a standstill, while Gianni is the first to raise concern about the economic situation, a concern made heavier by his responsibilities as an entrepreneur.

Antonio brings his humor to the table, urging others to consider that this is the time of those people, like him, who are used to being regarded as unsociable, as "bears." Suddenly, Luca falls ill, he seems to have contracted the virus: communication comes to a halt when, with a high fever, he is at the hospital waiting for a diagnosis and we are reunited in a group session.

Elena's mother passes away: the world and its tragedies cross the borders of our little group.

In the space of these two months the bonds between us have become very strong and emotional closeness is paramount: it is as if we all belonged to the same elective family. During the next few sessions we witness live Luca's healing process and the relief for the negative result of the test. Finally, he is released from isolation and can go back to having close contacts and physical demonstrations of affection, and we are moved by the hug with his grandmother.

The body in online group therapy

In another group, composed at the moment by seven people and led by two therapists, everyone joined the online sessions since day one of the lockdown.

Dina (45 years old) is a doctor and she's been fighting for a year against a particularly aggressive strain of breast cancer. In the last few months before the pandemic hit, she couldn't come to group therapy because she is immunodeficient and suffering a great deal from the heavy chemotherapy treatment. In this new situation created by the Covid-19 emergency, in which we were all quarantined in our homes and could communicate only on the phone or through the Internet, Dina has been able to safely participate in group therapy once again. One evening she shares with the group her anger at herself for getting sick and having to suffer through the therapy's side effects. She says she thinks it is kind of her fault that she fell ill because she has never gotten enough rest, she has always worked too much and she doesn't love herself. She is distressed because she thinks she "caused" her own tumor. She says she also feels the need to undertake a somatic therapy to give voice to her body, which she had repressed for too long.

Emilio (40 years old, engineer), who's usually withdrawn and obsessive, listens to her and is moved to tears. He asks Dina if she has noticed his heartfelt reaction while listening and she confirms that she has seen it and is shocked by it.

Cesare (53 years old, office worker) also participates in the conversation with feeling, reminding Dina that they are all there to support her.

Serena (48 years old, educator) agrees, while Mary (26 years old, psychologist) adds that she has to make it a priority, right now, to take care of herself. Laura (58 years old, pharmacist) has always felt very connected with Delia and she reminds her of when they both shared, during a group session, the fact that they hadn't felt welcomed and understood by their respective parents, telling her: "We aren't good at protecting ourselves, you

210

and me, we're learning just now." Dina starts trembling, tears streaming down her face, says her body is feeling a lot of different emotions and she feels everyone very close, as if in an embrace.

Everybody's emotional experience, including our therapists, is as truly deep and physical as if we were all in the same room.

Conclusions

The strong, emotionally intense experience we are going through can certainly be influenced by the socio-cultural climate in which the pandemic has plunged us: collective fears, generalized anxiety, diffidence, and need to trust, connect, and belong. It is a condition so close and current that, for now, it can't be read though the objectivity and neutrality of history. What we can say is that we are certain of the unique and exceptional nature of the present moment. It is possible, then, that the emotional openness we are observing and living may be a result of this extraordinary social situation. Certainly, we are surprised to note that the groups do work and that people are willing to go online and learn new ways of communicating in group too. After our initial surprise, observing the group, we could confirm that the essence of transactional exchanges in this setting is composed of language and the emotional connection passing, thanks to a visual connection, from our body to other people's, despite the lack of direct tactile contact. Words and transactions are not lost in an online setting and now technology allows us to establish visual contact with all members' corporeal presence at the same time (Chrome extensions like GridView are an example). Beyond words or images, the phantasmic presence of the Other is always alive and well in our minds and dreams. Thus, in some ways, online groups can assist in the creation of an oneiric environment which facilitates transference processes and allows passage – useful to the deconfusion process – between the social and the intrapsychic world.

As far as therapy is concerned, this experiment born out of necessity might take us in interesting research directions. The computer screen and the virtual connection grant us swift entrance into clients' inner worlds, removing barriers and inhibitions built in the familiar world of "in person" interactions, where our script apparatus was defined and where our defenses were first structured against the dangers that the Other can pose to ourselves.

Notes

1 For more on this, see: Retrieved June 22, 2020, from https://ec.europa.eu/digital-single-market/en/desi.
2 CNOP, the Italian National Council of the Order of Psychologists, created a database on its website to find a psychologist online for the first time on March 24, 2020. See: Retrieved October 20, 2020, from www.psy.it/psicologionline-la-professione-psicologica-a-disposizione-dei-cittadini.html.

References

American Medical Association. (2000). *Guidelines for patient–physician electronic mail.* Chicago: Author.

American Psychological Association. (1997). *APA statement on services by telephone, teleconferencing, and internet: A statement by the ethics committee of the American Psychological Association.* Washington, DC: Author.

American Psychological Association. (2012). *New generation of virtual humans helping to train psychologists.* Washington, DC: Author.

American Telemedicine Association. (2009a). *Evidence-based practice for telemental health.* Washington, DC: Author.

American Telemedicine Association. (2009b). *Practice guidelines for videoconferencing-based telemental health.* Washington, DC: Author.

American Telemedicine Association. (2010). *US states.* Washington, DC: Author.

Backhaus, A., Agha, Z., Maglione, M. L., Repp, A., Ross, B., Zuest, D., . . . Thorp, S. R. (2012). Videoconferencing psychotherapy: A systematic review. *Psychological Services, 9*(2), 111–131. doi:10.1037/a0027924

Baron, S. (2018). Online group psychotherapy: Ethical and legal issues. In S. S. Fehr (Ed.), *Introduction to group psychotherapy: A practical guide* (3rd ed., pp. 275–282). New York: Routledge Press.

Fehr, S. S. (2018). *Introduction to group psychotherapy: A practical guide* (3rd ed.). New York: Routledge Press.

Norwood, C., Moghaddam, N. G., Malins, S., & Sabin-Farrell, R. (2018). Working alliance and outcome effectiveness in videoconferencing psychotherapy: A systematic review and noninferiority meta-analysis. *Clinical Psychology & Psychotherapy, 25*(6), 797–808. doi:10.1002/cpp.2315

20

EFFICACY AND LIMITS OF GROUP PSYCHOTHERAPY

Transversal aspects of success

We saw how the feelings of loneliness and isolation, typical of European and North-American societies, render group setting particularly useful when it comes to healing and the stimulation of growth and empowerment in general. Emotional skills improve during sessions of group training, which often become psycho-educational workshops. In group, people learn how to communicate, recognize, and express their emotions and deal with conflict in a constructive way. They can also learn mediation strategies, persuasion, and influencing techniques. People who want to be empowered at work improve their techniques of public speaking and selling skills, often turn to group coaching.

Group therapy has different goals than coaching and professional training, since its objectives have more to do with care and the client's health. People who decide to embark in a therapeutic treatment expect results such as a deeper aware-ness and stable, structural change. Generally, people who choose group therapy can have two reasons: they either feel so bad they know they need a deeper kind of treatment, which the therapist usually suggests in their individual sessions; or they have the ambition to want for themselves a more firm and meaningful growth. Landaiche (2013, p. 296), building on the contributions of several TA scholars, pinpoints emotional education as the major takeaway of the group experience:

> The knowledge transmitted in an emotional education . . . comes indi-rectly, seeping through the cracks of the windowpanes, from under the floorboards and through the vents.
>
> (Brooks, 2009, p. 9)

When Newton (2003) wrote, "Transactional analysis began as a group therapy and to a certain extent it still is" (p. 321), she pointed to Berne's (1961) characterization of transactional analysis as an "indigenous approach derived from the group situation itself" (p. 165). Newton was also referencing an aspect of the transactional analysis tradition in which

DOI: 10.4324/9781003215547-21

significant emotional learning is seen as fundamental to the work in any group promoting learning, growth, and the recovery of what Berne (1964) called the capacities for "awareness, spontaneity and intimacy."(p. 178)

Limits of therapy

When group therapy fails to offer the expected result there might be several reasons. It was not the right time, the client is not motivated, the group is not stimulating enough, the therapist is not prepared enough to deal with the complex dynamics and tends to over adapt to members. Each one of these elements deserves to be analyzed and understood thoroughly.

Above all, it is important that, when suggesting a group, the therapist knows what they are doing. They need to have a solid working strategy and a clear idea of the context they are asking the client to join. It is also fundamental that the client is involved in the preparations and understands the journey they are being asked to embark upon. Pre-group preparation and the contract are crucial first moments and must be taken into account through the whole shared journey. Additionally, the group needs to be involved in the contracting process of each member's goal. The group itself acts as co-therapist. A group that is too passive and detached does not facilitate affiliation or change. The difficulty in setting up a therapy or educational group lies precisely in the search for a dynamic balance between the safety the group provides and the challenges born out of discomfort and of the need to find new ways to adjust.

There are moments, occasionally long stretches of time, when we live our professional lives in the grip of our personal histories. At the unconscious heart of each one of us, there are deep echoes, shadows, voices from the past that are still very much alive in the present and often shape and twist the way we see the world, what we want and the way we treat others. These profoundly formative experiences, phantoms and desires date back to our childhoods, and often remain in the way we are for the rest of our lives, also emerging unconsciously in the course of the therapeutic relationship. This is true for both client and therapist.

The specific technique of TA

Transactional analysis was born precisely as a group therapy, and many transactional analysts' clients employ group therapy as primary therapy model.

In group, TA deals with explicit transactions and the way a set of transactions act during a session. Every behavior is observed and analyzed as expression of an internal dialogue (structural analysis of the ego states) and as stimulus within a stimulus-answer system (transactional analysis proper). The concepts of TA become, in time, an element of group culture.

According to a great group analyst, the main traits of a TA group (Moiso, 1998) may be summarized as such:

1   Active involvement of the therapist;
2   Existence of specific contracts regarding both procedure and content of therapy, including clinical objectives. Contract does not merely mean an agreed-upon objective, but the definition of the setting, in particular when it comes to the commitment between therapist and members and between members themselves. Each member will be required to define their own goals, independently from their metacognitive skills. This helps the client understand what they need, allows the definition of roles and boundaries, and encourages a collaborative participation from all clients. Members also commit to express thoughts and emotional experiences tied to what happens in group, in order to facilitate a climate of intimacy and spontaneity;
3   Implementation of a well-planned therapeutic strategy through stages of analysis, redecision, reparenting, and reelaboration;
4   Use of delineated and sequential contact tactics and therapeutic intervention strategies apt for the different types of clients (strategy represents the direction toward a goal, while tactic refers to the modes of operation);
5   Practice of specific therapeutic operations;
6   Therapy work involving, on the one hand, the socio-behavioral level, and on the other, dynamic and intrapsychic aspects;
7   A personalized definition of healing in both operative and existential terms.

In the previous chapters, we have described the characteristics of therapeutic planning, the strategic choices, and the intervention techniques.

The possibility of employing group psychotherapy with very different clients and contracts built on the individual and their needs allows the client to work at the same time on a cognitive level – to improve self-awareness and uncover the mental traps that sometimes keep them so unhappy – and on an emotional level – to learn basic emotional skills and live reparative coping experiences. For those who wish to work on a deeper level, the group is also a psychodynamic environment of emotional regression, transference projections, and scrip redecision.

Additionally, transactional analysis counts among its main features the use of the group as a space for the education and learning of professionals.

The group is first and foremost experience, then object of study, and space of supervision and feedback in the processes of examination and international affiliation to recognized associations such as ITAA and EATA.

215

How to train a group therapist

We know that the training of transactional analysts and group therapists takes many years to be completed. It is structured differently according to the country in which people are trained and the different legislations on the matter, but all professional communities have established very high standards in terms of number of hours of training, internship, supervision, and professional practice.

Those who work in this field are aware of the steps they have to go through with their trainees and know that any kind of training must include a personal experience of individual and group therapy, as well as constant supervision in the course of their entire professional practice.

Yalom (2005), in a relevant study on the matter, delineates the fundamental guidelines in the training of a group therapist: "(1) Observation of experienced group therapists at work; (2) close clinical supervision of trainees' maiden groups; (3) a personal group experience; and (4) personal psychotherapeutic work" (Yalom & Leszcz, 2005, p. 670). Our model of work follows these guidelines closely.

In a marvelous and bold article, Baba Neal (2017) argues:

> This brings me to the issue of psychotherapy training. There are certain myths about psychotherapists that are unwittingly created and maintained by our general reluctance to discuss openly our vulnerabilities, mistakes, and failures. These discussions need to be modeled in training, with experienced therapists normalizing troubling aspects of our experience as psychotherapists. Maintaining "the myth of the untroubled therapist" (Adams, 2004, p. 4) and of the ever-successful therapy is costly at many levels: It stops us from seeking help, it stops us from acting with compassion, and it creates unrealistic standards and oppressive taboos against which new generations of therapists struggle.
>
> Sussman (1995) argued that part of the education of astronauts and firefighters is an "appreciation of the dangers that they will face" (p. 2), but most prospective psychotherapists go into this work unaware that there is a dark underbelly to psychotherapy practice.
>
> (Baba Neal, 2017, p. 179)

The training institution is the first example to a trainee of how groups may work in a healthy or pathological manner. Training begins in the institution where trainees have to attend a period of individual therapy, training analysis in group and seminars divided up in classes that work as groups. The very teaching staff works in groups and the organization of the institution shares several traits with small groups. In a famous work titled *Ideology, Conflict, and Leadership in Groups and Organizations*, Otto Kernberg (1998) described how ideologies, conflicts, and leadership styles also appear within psychoanalytic institutions.

Still relevant today is the description of the four organizational models that institutions can aspire to – art academy, technical trade school, theological seminary or religious retreat, and a college at a university – so as the suggestion to combine the college with the art academy model.

The most fragile trainees, as the most vulnerable clients, constitute a precious resource when questioning the models employed by institutions and psychotherapies: they show us where our systems fail and we should be grateful to them because they push us to be better.

Supervision

Often, colleagues look for a supervisor when they are having trouble, feel on the brink of a professional crisis or burned-out. It is obviously advisable that a therapist ask for help when they feel like they need it, but it would be more useful to choose a permanent support and formative figure.

In TA training, we consider supervision a constant exchange with a senior therapist who is certified to be able to provide formative support to their colleagues. Our training programs are marked by international exams which represent a real initiation and affiliation ritual. The titles of supervisor and teacher are the most coveted and are achieved after several years of training and a series of exams.

Much has been written on supervision in TA. Marco Mazzetti (2007) won the Berne prize for his article in which he looks at the philosophy and method behind supervision in TA. Among the most recent contributions on this topic, the most relevant is Helena Hargaden's (2016) text on the art of group supervision. The group is the central element of all five stages of the relational approach to supervision: clinical presentation, group process as answer to the presentation, reflection of the group on the group process, and theoretical perspectives in dialogue with the professional presenting the case.

Again, we can see here the emergence of "the Third," as treated in previous chapters from Benjamin's perspective.

Hargaden writes:

> The third refers to the creation of a triangular symbolic space which can emerge from a collision polarities in which a third ways is formed. . . . The relational third is most frequently associated with an intersubjective perspective. . . . It refers to an innate sense of self with other that we bring to every meeting: it is the process by which we share experience with each other both consciously and unconsciously.
>
> (2016, p. 24)

Working in group on supervision improves professionals' possibilities of receiving essential formative stimuli to become group therapists and strengthen their skills in the handling of dynamics and processes.

Baba Neal, in the previously mentioned article, writes about the necessity to learn from our problems and failures. In her case, from the experience of a client's suicide:

> The association between trauma and initiation – which is meant to be a memorable rite of transition – makes sense. Pain, suffering, and fear are emotions that mediate a learning that becomes permanently encoded in the brain. We learn things more easily and retain them longer if they are associated with intense emotion.
>
> Most transactional analysis practitioners would probably identify the Certified Transactional Analyst (CTA) and the Teaching and Supervising Transactional Analyst (TSTA) exams and the rituals involved as proxy for traumatic initiation. However, I consider my true initiation into the profession to have occurred unexpectedly and prematurely at the time of Aria's death. Her suicide showed me the darker, wounding aspects of my chosen profession, which had not even been hinted at previously. This experience forced me to demythologize my role (Pope, Sonne, & Greene, 2006). . . . Given the stigma that has surrounded suicide at many times, it is not surprising that therapists experience strong negative countertransference to their suicidal clients (Maltsberger & Buie, 1974) ranging from indifference or pity to anger, sadism, malice, and contempt. At the same time, our professional self-esteem is predicated on feeling caring, compassionate, and nonjudgmental. In this context, accepting and confessing to punitive and rejecting feelings is risky. Maltzberger and Buie believe that accepting our negative countertransference can reduce our tendency to act out in ways that convey to the client "I do not want to be with you" because such ruptures in the therapeutic relationship with a suicidal client can have severe consequences.
>
> I have learned to accept myself at those times when I am stirred by negative countertransference and I lose my patience and compassion. I think it is inevitable that working with clients who are empathically disconnected from themselves and others will create a style of interaction that is unpredictable and turbulent. When I accept that turbulence as part of the process, I am less likely to hold on to an idealized vision of the psychotherapeutic endeavor and more accepting of myself and my limitations. I can be more flexible and creative in my interventions when I accept that I will make mistakes and that it is important to own up when I have done so. Perhaps, at some level, clients pick up that I am robust, resilient, and unafraid to walk down some dark alleys.
>
> (2017, pp. 10–11)

Only a personal reelaboration of the therapist's trauma through personal therapy and supervision might allow them to reach the maturity and richness we find in Baba Neal.

The ethics of group work

The therapist's ethical approach is comprised first of all of the honesty and clarity they employ in the communication with their clients and the group as a whole, as well as their responsibility for their own competence or incompetence.

To be in an ethical and fair position toward the group means above all not keeping secrets from clients, allowing everyone to be in a space that promotes equity and well-being, and knowing when to let clients go when it is clear that moving forward will not be of any help.

There are cases in which closing the group might be the best solution, especially if supervision confirms that the space is no longer healing for its members.

In a case we have followed as supervisors, two therapists had been co-leading a group for four years. The dynamic between them had become dysfunctional because unconsciously competitive and, because each one also led other groups without their co-therapist, they always ended up inserting new clients only in the groups they led individually. Thus, the co-led group had trouble moving forward, and the two were not telling each other that they were letting the group die because they could not communicate properly. Supervision brought to light the underlying dynamics and the two decided for an amicable "divorce" after finishing up their work with their common clients. Nonetheless, after having made this explicit between them and having come to this decision, which was not communicated to the group, the clients' position changed radically, since they seemed to wake up after an endless stillness. From that moment on, they started making more of an effort and the group ended with successful outcomes for all members.

In an interesting article on the failure of therapy, William Cornell writes about the way transference and countertransference dynamics become quicksand in which both therapist and clients sink when enactments are so powerful they cause the therapist to lose their capacity for reflection:

When the professional can create a reflective space, clients have a better opportunity to see and gradually become free of their scripts. But with Samantha I was affected in such powerful ways that I could not hold my reactions in consciousness. I could not make sense of my own experience. There were aspects of myself and my personal history that were called into a compelling (though unconscious) being, which I found unbearable. The result was a contradictory and inconsistent combination of my feeling overly responsible, avoidant, and compliant. Without some clarity and distance from my side of the relationship, it became impossible for Samantha to step out of her transferential reactions and demands on me. We became blinded in the dark shadows of our pasts.

(p. 6)

It is a matter of professional ethics to commit to being competent and seek competence, and it is also a matter of ethics to recognize our ignorance in certain fields and maintain a position of true commitment toward our clients, keeping greed and narcissism – a therapist's two main demons – in check.

Our possible influence on others might stroke our narcissism and our feeling of being almighty might be reinforced by an adoring group. But an honest therapist knows that group conformism might mislead us and we should not always be satisfied when people act with complacency toward us.

In the aforementioned article, which contains a deep, honest analysis of therapeutic failure and the restoration of reflective capacity as one of the therapist's responsibilities, Cornell (2016) adds:

Within relational models lay both gratification and potential danger within the therapeutic dyad. The therapeutic relationship offers both client and therapist an unusual sense of intimacy and exclusivity. It is a protected relationship that offers a unique and compelling kind of closeness. But it is a closeness that needs to end, that needs to be a temporary foundation that lays the ground for clients to move out into the world. Most of the time, there is an inherent developmental pressure within the therapeutic process that moves the client out toward the world at large. Most of the time, the experience of the therapeutic work itself creates a space that challenges the comfort of the therapeutic dyad. But when the therapist and client become locked in an effort to compensate for the pain and losses of childhood, an unhealthy symbiosis forms that can offer comfort and predictability but cuts off the development of emotional maturity, personal agency, and true intimacy.

(pp. 7–8)

There are clients who disappear angrily from groups and who can teach a lot to both therapist and members, as we have seen in Chapter 17 on the end of therapy. The ethical approach adds to this analysis a respect of the Other's freedom and the acknowledgment of their reasons, however mad they might seem to the group, which, akin to a small society, would prefer conformity in order to feel safe.

The group in education, coaching, and counseling

We have not discussed the use of the group in the fields of counseling and education. Transactional analysis has an excellent track record in all such fields of application, deserving of another volume altogether.

Patrizia Vinella is one of the most competent TSTA in her field. Her 2013 contribution is considered a reference point in recent theory and practice of group counseling. As she clearly states:

> The main objectives of a counseling group are improving communication among group members, developing awareness of communication styles (stroke economy, transactions, games, drivers), facilitating the expression and management of emotions (Cornell & Hine, 1999), developing clients' resources, and preventing distress. The leader facilitates the exchange of opinions among group members. What emerges from such exchanges, in accordance with the counseling contract, is shared with the others in an Adult-oriented process. This aspect is easier when the contract has been clearly defined and involves common goals. The change process is thus delineated around a central problem shared by all group members. The group focus therefore becomes "care rather than cure."
>
> (Loomis, 1982, p. 52; Vinella, 2013, p. 70)

Vinella believes that the counseling group differs from the psychotherapy group in several elements such as goals, but also contracts, methods, and duration:

> I have observed that the elements that enhance the definition of a group contract are having a group that is homogeneous, closed, and time limited.
>
> The term homogeneous refers to the clients themselves and not to the problems they may have (e.g., they are all parents, elderly people, adolescents, teachers, etc.). Berne (1966, p. 5) wrote that with therapy groups, it was best to choose patients randomly or in any way that would make the group as heterogeneous as possible in terms of the pathologies that needed to be addressed. In counseling groups, homogeneity is preferable because then common goals for change are easier to find.
>
> Homogeneity makes it easier to establish a group contract and facilitates communication among group members. In a closed group the participants remain the same from the beginning to the end, which favors cohesion among members and the growth of the group as a whole.
>
> A limit to the duration of the group (e.g., 6–10 meetings of 2–3 hours each) leads to a clearer definition of the group boundaries and the development of a counseling work plan.
>
> (p. 72)

In our opinion, this setting appears more appropriate to group therapy with children and teenagers because it has a more defined duration in time and it can be employed with members belonging to the same age group.

Therapy groups for children and teenagers

We have preferred not to mention groups for children and under-aged teenagers, since the topic is beyond the scope of this exposition. Discussing the treatment of children in TA, Gjurković and Tudor (2018) led us to understand how a group dimension is present in the work between therapist, parents and children.

> Working with children always involves a three-handed contract between the child, the parent(s)/caregiver(s), and the therapist
>
> (Tudor, 2008).

> When working with children (depending on their age), this stage is characterized by the exploratory use of the playroom, toys, and (board) games through which the child becomes more familiar with the therapist and learns what to expect from her or him (Norton & Norton, 2006). Mutual trust starts to grow during this stage, and the child may gain some social control of his or her dysfunctional behaviors. In the parallel psychoeducative/counseling process with parents, it is also of great importance to establish a working alliance. This provides feelings of safety and trust, the parents become much more engaged in the process, and the fantasy that the "therapist will fix my child's problems" diminishes.
>
> (pp. 3–4)

Dolores Munari Poda (2004, 2018), too, stresses the group aspect inherent in working with children:

> A child is a group – in the sense of an amalgam of affects, conditioning, complexity, and relationships – a relational system and a vital system.
>
> Those who work with children in any capacity need a particularly stable physical and psychic balance.
>
> The attention to the group and the environment must be steadfast. It is necessary to be able to communicate with ancient and new emotions. It is necessary to be familiar with one's own existential journey and one's own inner Child, and it is important to recognize one's own vulnerability.
>
> We always meet the child and their family in a relational perspective which sees the therapist involved first-hand in a creative project of which all concerned parties are aware: child, therapist, family, reference group.
>
> (Munari Poda, 2018, p. 31)

Additionally, Stefano Morena and colleagues write, in a soon to be published article:

> In complex traumatic situations, individual psychotherapy is a necessary condition for recovery, but it is insufficient, not enough: In fact, it is necessary to reactivate/rebuild a group that functions as family or as an alternative to family, which would offer the child or the adolescent an alphabet useful to analyze, re-read and process what happens to them. To be wounded is not only the individual but also the community to which they belong. If trauma hits a collectivity, its processing also needs to take place within a group. For this reason, it is crucial to work on both levels: individual and group.
>
> (Morena, Spinelli, & Bergamaschi, 2021)

Many TA therapists experience group therapy with children and teenagers, but not much has been yet written on the potential of group work with TA in the pediatric age.

In our work experience with children and adolescents at school, group work was used in the curricula of health education as a psychoeducational activity promoting circle-time. In circle-time, children learn how to recognize their emotions, verbalize, and communicate them in a constructive way to others, and are involved in games aimed at improving self-knowledge (Tangolo, 1991). Such activities, which may be more related to the fields of education and counseling, have nonetheless a strong therapeutic impact on the most ailing and troubled children.

In a circle-time group, Filippo, 12 years old, never spoke, as he was suffering from selective mutism also the whole time he was in school. One day, after being asked to by one of the facilitators, he wrote on a piece of paper: I am a child without friends and that's why I can hear the trees speak.

The facilitator received the paper and asked permission to read Filippo's message aloud to the group. Filippo agreed and from that moment on, the group listened to Filippo's words, which he kept writing poetically on paper at first, and then started to express vocally to the others.

Quiet Filippo translated to his fellow members the words of trees and woods, and by doing so he started to speak and play with other humans again. We could say that Filippo healed from selective mutism without any specific psychotherapy treatment, but within the therapeutic context of circle-time, which he attended at school and which was conducted with transactional analysis techniques.

On this matter, Anna Emanuela adds:

> *In my experience as a school psychologist, I encountered hundreds of groups of children from 11 to 18 years old, and I believe I learned a lot as a therapist for adults. I learned how a child suffers and feels left out, how difficult it might be for them to be accepted and welcomed in a new group, how essential the others' recognition of a success or virtue becomes in order to feel good about themselves. For the youngest, the group is fundamental. If you have a group in which to grow up, you can blossom and find out who you really are.*

Thus, much has yet to be written on transactional analysis groups in the pediatric age.

Conclusions

We are publishing this book 50 years after Eric Berne's death and we find the international community of transactional analysis to be a rather lively and prolific environment, open to research and contamination by neuroscientific and relational psychology studies.

In the words of Willian Cornell (2020) from a recent study of his:

> Our clients, students, supervisees, and colleagues certainly need structure and recognition, but when that comes at the cost of stimulation, uncertainty, difference, and curiosity, our work becomes impoverished.
>
> Our most difficult patients challenge our narcissism as well as our ways of thinking and working. It is then through our conversations and consultations with each other as professionals with the capacity to be interested in our differences, the capacity to recognize the limits of our models as well as their strengths, that our work stays alive. We, as professionals, stay alive and have the flexibility and capacity to engage with a truly broad range of people. Then our clients, students, supervisees, and colleagues also have the freedom to be themselves.
>
> (p. 176)

We believe group therapists should be constantly open to listening, knowledge, and interaction with their present's culture. We believe it useful to learn everyday what makes us human, ever more human, part of a plural collectivity. Group therapists can count on Group therapists can count on clients' knowledge, their ability to challenge themselves, and the spontaneous interest pushing us all toward each other, pushing us all toward a We.

Thus, we can confirm that during this writing journey we have indeed learned a lot from clients, colleagues and trainees. That is the meaning of journey we wanted to share throughout the book, a journey in the land of theory and transformative practice, two elements indissolubly intertwined offering new spaces and territories to explore. We are grateful to this journey and we will without a doubt continue along this path.

References

Adams, M. (2004). *The myth of the untroubled therapist: Private life, professional practice*. London and New York: Routledge.

Baba Neal, S. (2017). The impact of a client's suicide. *Transactional Analysis Journal*, *47*(3), 173–185. doi:10.1177/0362153717711701

Berne, E. (1961). *Transactional analysis in psychotherapy: A systematic individual and social psychiatry*. New York: Grove Press.

Berne, E. (1964). *Games people play: The psychology of human relationships*. New York: Grove Press.

Berne, E. (1966). *Principles of group treatment*. Oxford: Oxford University Press.

Brooks, D. (2009). The other education. *International Herald Tribune, 9*.

Cornell, W. F. (2016). Failing to do the job: When the client pays the price for the therapist's countertransference. *Transactional Analysis Journal*, *46*(4), 266–276. doi:10.1177/0362153716661719

Cornell, W. F. (2020). Transactional analysis and psychoanalysis: Overcoming the narcissism of small differences in the shadow of Eric Berne. *Transactional Analysis Journal*, *50*(3), 164–178. doi:10.1080/03621537.2020.1771020

Cornell, W. F., & Hine, J. (1999). Cognitive and social functions of emotions: A model for transactional analysis counselor training. *Transactional Analysis Journal*, *29*(3), 175–185. doi:10.1177/036215379902900303

Gjurković, T., & Tudor, K. (2018). Treatment stages in working with children: An approach rooted in transactional analysis and play therapy. *Transactional Analysis Journal*, *48*(3), 242–257. doi:10.1080/03621537.2018.1471291

Hargaden, H. (Ed.). (2016). *The art of relational supervision: Clinical implications of the use of self in group supervision*. New York and London: Routledge.

Kernberg, O. F. (1998). *Ideology, conflict, and leadership in groups and organizations*. New Haven, CT: Yale University Press.

Landaiche, N. M. (2013). Looking for trouble in groups developing the professional's capacity. *Transactional Analysis Journal*, *43*(4), 296–310. doi:10.1177/0362153713516296

Loomis, M. (1982). Contracting for change. *Transactional Analysis Journal*, *12*, 51–54. doi:10.1177/036215378201200107

Maltsberger, J. T., & Buie, D. H. (1974). Countertransference hate in the treatment of suicidal patients. *Archives of General Psychiatry*, *30*(5), 625–633.

Mazzetti, M. (2007). Supervision in transactional analysis an operational model. *Transactional Analysis Journal*, *37*(2), 93–103. doi:10.1177/036215370703700202

Moiso, C. (1998). Il setting in psicoterapia di gruppo. In M. Novellino (Ed.), *L'approccio clinico dell'analisi transazionale*. Milano: Franco Angeli.

Morena, S., Spinelli, M., & Bergamaschi, M. (2021). *Genitori, Bambini e Adolescenti nella Pandemic. Dalla Ricercar all'Intervento Clinico*. Neopsiche. Rivets di A.T. e Scienze Umane, 30. Unpublished manuscript.

Munari Poda, D. (2004). Every child is a group: The girl of the snakes. *Transactional Analysis Journal, 34*(1), 52–68. doi:10.1177/036215370403400107

Munari Poda, D. (2018). *Ciao, ti stave aspettando. L'incontro clinico con ill bambino* (Vol. I). Brescia: Serra Tarantola Editore.

Newton, T. (2003). Identifying educational philosophy and practice through imagoes in transactional analysis training groups. *Transactional Analysis Journal, 33*(4), 321–331. doi:10.1177/036215370303300407

Norton, C. C., & Norton, B. E. (2006). Experiential play therapy. In C. E. Schaefer & H. G. Kaduson (Cur.), *Contemporary play therapy* (pp. 28–54). New York: Guilford.

Pope, K. S., Sonne, J. L., & Greene, B. (2006). *What therapists don't talk about and why: Understanding taboos that hurt us and our clients*. Washington, DC: American Psychological Association.

Sussman, M. B. (1995). *A perilous calling: The hazards of psychotherapy practice*. New York: Wiley.

Tudor, K. (2008). Working with the individual child using transactional analysis. In K. Tudor (Ed.), *The adult is parent to the child: Transactional analysis with children and young people* (pp. 89–103). Lyme Regis: Russell House.

Vinella, P. (2013). Transactional analysis counseling groups: Theory, practice, and how they differ from other TA groups. *Transactional Analysis Journal, 43*(1), 68–79. doi:10.1177/0362153713486111

Yalom, I. D., & Leszcz, M. (2005). *The theory and practice of group psychotherapy* (5th ed.). New York: Basic Books (Originally published in 1970).

APPENDIX

The concept of ego states is widely used in transactional analysis to explain the basis of the functioning of the mind and human behaviors. An ego state is a mixture of cognitive representations, emotions and models of behaviors, all related to each other.

We can say that our minds express thousands of ego states in the course of our lives.

The concept of Parent, Adult and Child are attempts to simplify and categorize mind states that go through an evolutionary organization during our development. Thus, in an effort to make more accessible to everyone several complex ideas described in this book, we have decided to provide a synthetic representation of the aforementioned development in terms of the PAC model.

Group psychotherapy provides a valuable experience that facilitates the integration of the clients' split parts, so as to improve mirroring in others and recover as adults those emotional connections the most fragile clients lacked during their childhood.

Psychoevolutionary development

We shall try to delineate in a synthetic manner the evolutionary stages that mark an individual's personality organization according to the transactional analytic approach.

In describing the evolutionary levels of the ego states the nomenclature defines as level 0 the level of psychic organization of the individual; level 1, the level of psychic evolution anchored to emotional memory and the child's pre-logic intuitive thought; level 2, the level of language acquisition and second-order thought. Each level of development contains the previous ones.

In this chapter, we shall describe the development of the Adult's (A_2) ability to reflect on their own ego states as well as others', and recognize themselves as psychic agents, able to think and act (Fonagy, Gergely, Jurist, & Target, 2002).

From birth to the sixth/seventh month of their life, the newborn's personality structure in AT is called the Somatic Child and it is composed of C_0, A_0 e P_0.

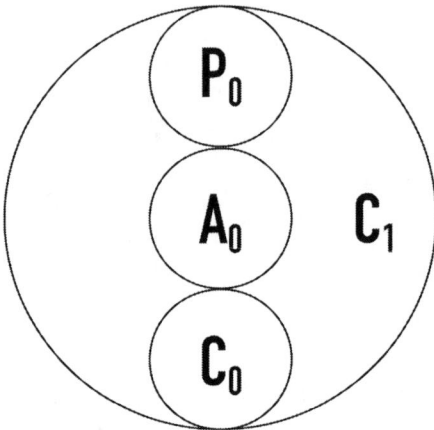

During this time, moving in the surrounding space, the newborn learns that their actions produce certain changes in this space and allow them to differentiate their bodily self from the outside world. They manifest an innate propension to interact affectively with their caregivers, imitating facial expressions and sharing their emotional and intentional states. Such interactive exchanges between caregiver and child of an early age imply the existence of a "primary intersubjectivity" which "functions as a mechanism for attributing intentional, motivational, and feeling states to the other during early imitative interactions" (Fonagy et al., 2002, p. 211).

From the sixth month to the second year of life, a structure called Little Professor, or A_1 starts to develop.

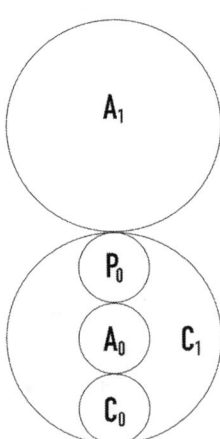

The Little Professor is able to discriminate their actions on the basis of their consequences, and choose the most effective way to reach a target starting from a set of options. This constitutes the intuitive, creative and curious part of the child's personality. During this time, the child learns a series of "joint-attention skills" (Fonagy et al., 2002) thanks to which they employ communicative gestures in order to direct the adults' attention toward objects or situations. As Novellino and Moiso (1982) remind us, the child, after having discovered, in the former stage, that they exist, and that their actions produce change in the external environment and in others, begins to understand how things work.

From the second to third year of their life, a P_1 is formed, also called Electrode, in order to highlight the automatism of their responses to external stimuli, an automatism which contains the permissions and prohibitions coming from the educational figures surrounding the child.

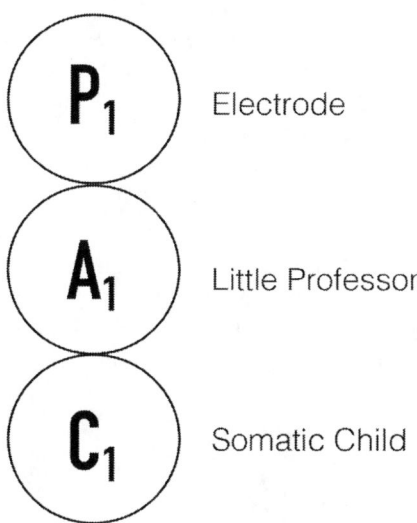

P_1 — Electrode

A_1 — Little Professor

C_1 — Somatic Child

The P_1 represents the internalized external object which might or might not satisfy the needs of the C_1. When such needs are satisfied, the child will experience the introjected object as having a positive polarity (P_{1+}), as opposed to when the need fails to be satisfied, and the object will be experienced as having a negative polarity (P_{1-}) (Miglionico & Novellino, 1993). If the relational experiences with caregivers are good enough, the child will be able to overcome the ambivalence of P_{1+} and P_{1-}, with the subsequent fusion of the two into a definitive P_1.

At this age, the child starts to have language to express emotions, experiences an interest toward other people's feelings and desires. They are now able to distinguish between their own and others' desires and, as a consequence, the Little Professor might mediate between C_0's and the caregivers' needs. If, for example, parents do not approve expressions of painful emotions such as tears or complaints, the Little Professor will elaborate a strategy so as to clam up and stop manifesting such emotions, and, in the long run, might incorporate in their P_1 the automatism of not asking for help when they are in trouble. Thus, in their adult life, they will automatically react to painful events denying themselves emotional outbursts and cries for help (Novellino & Moiso, 1982).

The ability – acquired at this age – of regulating emotions and tolerating frustrations thanks to their mirroring relationship with their caregivers allows the Little Professor to modulate C_0's impulses, adapting them to the interactive context. This happens when the child perceives that their attachment figures think about them and considers them other, different from their own person, a mental and intentional agent with individual traits. This mirroring ability of the caregivers, that is, the ability to be in synch, to reflect and express the inner states the child manifests, constitutes the solid basis on which the child's A_1 may begin "mentalizing their emotions" and thus regulating C_1's affections: recognized feelings do not need to be acted out and can be shared. This way, the child will be able to reflect upon their emotions. Repeated experiences with significant others such as caregivers, siblings, grandparents, and teachers allow the child to assign them generalized intentions and attitudes which will become fixed traits in their representation of others, internalized in their P_2, which will form around eight years of age.

When the child is provided a healthy affective mirroring environment, at four years old the formation of the Child ego state is finally complete. This component of an individual's personality contains emotions, thoughts and behaviors which, in their adult life, will be associated with the self-realization function, the basis on which to build collaborative, creative and intimate social bonds (Temple, 1999). This personality component is called C_2, to distinguish it from the Somatic Child (C_1).

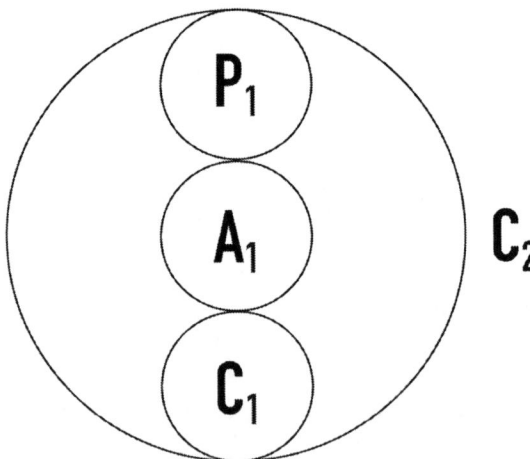

The integrated and integrating Adult, A_2 forms between four and six years of age, and possesses a coherent and unified autobiographical representation of self.

The sense of personal continuity allows the Adult to explore thoughts, feelings and behaviors belonging to Child and Parent, and adapt them to their experience of the present. The A_2 possesses the ability to mentalize, meaning the ability to understand others' actions, as well as its own, in terms of thoughts, feelings, hopes, and desires. Thanks to this ability, individuals can alter their script beliefs in light of new information and new stimuli from the outside world. It is in relation to this particular aspect, linked to an endless process of integration and alteration, that Temple (1999) introduced the concept of the integrating Adult. Referring to the Adult, Tudor (2003) defines it as "integrating" in order to highlight its critical and reflective awareness, as well as its motivational drives: "It is the capacity to reflect on ourselves and others, to spit out those experiences or introjections that are no longer relevant, and to assimilate the past in service of the present, that defines the 'Integrating Adult'" (p. 219).

The structuring of personality is complete around eight years of age through the energization of the Parent ego state, P_2, which differentiates itself from P_1 because it is introjected from the outside (Novellino & Moiso, 1982). It contains the set of thoughts, feelings and behaviors the child acquired from the caregivers and other formative figures in the first years of their life. Temple links this ego state to the social responsibility function, since it provides structures and care for themselves and others.

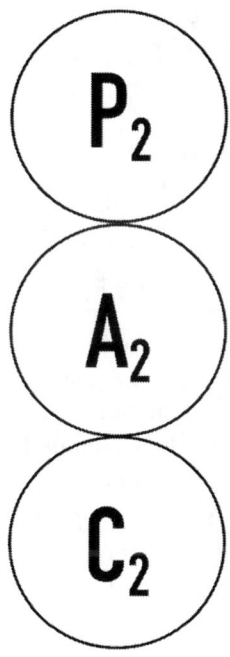

Psychopathologic development

As we have seen, the ability of the integrating and integrated Adult to find the multiple meanings of its own mind, as well as others', constitutes an intrapsychic, interpersonal evolutionary achievement which might be subject to conflict and defenses. This ability is developed during the early attachment relationships, when the caregivers' minds are mature, reflective and syntonic enough, or, simply put, when caregivers possess an integrating and integrated Adult.

If the child cannot see their own mental states represented in the other's mind, they will have to employ a good amount of resources in order to understand the caregiver's behavior, hindering their A_1's development of its own reflective thinking with regard to C_1's needs. In transactional analysis, this process is related to a lack of acceptance of the ambivalence of P_{1+} and P_{1-}, as well as a lack of integration in P_1, which we call the split P_1: The external object will be perceived alternatively as all "good" or all "bad." The split P_1, present in the borderline structure of personality, reveals a remarkable emotional instability that might involve, in turn, violent, impulsive manifestations (Miglionico & Novellino, 1993).

A caregiver who cannot perceive or metabolize the child's anxieties prevents them from gradually building a representation of their own inner states, thus keeping these in their minds and containing them. Fear and anger become parts of them, they cannot be thought and as such they become acted out against the other or the self. The external reality is confused with the internal one, A_1 cannot distinguish C_1's needs from P_1's, thus failing to confer meaning and coherence to their own actions.

In order to better explain this phenomenon, we can employ the concept of ego state relational unit elaborated by Little (2006). According to the author, Child and Parent are not considered as singular ego states but as relational unit categories which, in case of a failure in the relationship between child and caregiver, remain fixed and introjected in a system closed to the outside world. The relational symbiosis between child and caregiver then transforms into an inner symbiosis between a Persecutor Parent, intrusive and disagreeable, and an helpless victim Child, symbiosis which constitutes the destructive mechanism at the root of many symptoms of personality disorders. Those who suffer from such disorders employ their energies in keeping this inner conflict alive: remaining frozen in their traumatic childhood, they experience "too much" trauma and "too little" of the present time. The challenge of group therapy will be to help these personality organizations to integrate past memories within a coherent narrative – not "relived" but shared memories – restoring their ability to explore their internal and external reality through the eyes of the integrating and integrated Adult.

References

Fonagy, P., Gergely, G., Jurist, E. L., & Target, M. (2002). *Affect regulation, mentalization, and the development of the self.* New York: Other Press.

Little, R. (2006). Ego state relational units and resistance to change. *Transactional Analysis Journal, 36*(1), 7–19. doi:10.1177/036215370603600103

Miglionico, A., & Novellino, M. (1993). *Il Sé limite: Analisi transazionale psicodinamica e patologia di confine.* Milano: Franco Angeli.

Novellino, M., & Moiso, C. (1982). *Stati dell'Io.* Roma: Astrolabio.

Temple, S. (1999). Functional fluency for educational transactional analysis. *Transactional Analysis Journal, 29*(3), 164–174. doi:10.1177/036215379902900302

Tudor, K. (2003). The neopsyche: The integrating adult ego state. In H. Hargaden & C. Sills (Eds.), *Ego states: Key concepts in transactional analysis: Contemporary views* (pp. 201–231). London: Worth Publishing.

INDEX

Note: Page numbers in **bold** indicate a table on the corresponding page.